RESILIENCE: Successful Psychotherapies

By Peter Alan Olsson MD

Sometimes I ask myself why I ever chose *The Impossible Profession*(s) of psychiatry and psychoanalysis—then I recall my work with some interesting, resilient, and courageous young souls. As a psychiatrist psychotherapist for over forty years I found challenges, failures, rewards even joy, in my work. It was particularly meaningful to work with adults or youths who were curious and thoughtful about how their mind, relationships, and emotions could be effectively understood. I admired them when they genuinely embraced their therapy project to master their conflicts, resolve their fears, and eliminate their blind spots. As they grew in mindfulness, self-awareness and maturity, I felt privileged to be a part of their journey.

In this book, I describe a group of unique boys [Note: possibly "individuals" rather than "boys" because later in the narrative Juan Gomez is older and Howard Scott's story is concurrent with Davey Scott's story when Howard takes responsibility for his relapse.] I worked with in psychotherapy or encountered in my clinical work. Their stories are interesting and poignant but the characteristic most striking about them was their **resilience**. It was so necessary for success in their/our hard work of psychotherapy. I chose them to write about because of my admiration for their candor and resilience. Only one of them was severely psychotic and never got treatment. The rest of them all had significant issues necessary to master to move forward with success in their lives.

Each therapy involved my patients' families in significant ways and though cooperation by families was obviously important, it was not always possible or imperative for a positive [therapy result] outcome. I have carefully tried to protect the confidentiality of my patients by disguising places, names and some events. However, I believe the essence of their life stories and therapy process has been maintained. I have sought concision in the stories by condensing time periods and editing descriptions of lengthy intervals involving the fallowing of insights and the gradual working through of an insight or domain of mindfulness. I sometimes emphasize dramatic and important psychotherapy events by exact dialogue and descriptions. I hope these convey the essence of important psychotherapy work. At the end of each chapter I will describe what I learned from each [of my boys].

Unlike many melodramatic Hollywood movie scenarios, changes occurring in psychotherapy are often deceptively quiet, often muted. Psychotherapy involves many emotional experiences—anxiety, fear, fascination, wonder, boredom, humor/laughter, anger, sadness, and often pain. The more severe and ominous forms of pain, destruction, and even a death prevented, go unheralded. They are unnoticed because existentially they like a suicide prevented, never in fact exist or occur.

CONTENTS:

1—A BOY WHO LOVED KNIVES

2—A BOY WHO WATCHED HIS FATHER MURDERED

3—A BOY WHO DIDN'T TALK FOR 40 YEARS

4—A BOY NAMED TOMMY AND HIS TROUBLED MOM

5—A BOY WHO LONGED TO GO TO PRISON

6—A BOY WHO WAS A WOULD-BE BOMBER

7—A BOY WHO LOVED HIS CRAZY DAD [per note in introduction about Howard the title here could be— A BOY AND HIS CRAZY DAD

8—A BOY ABANDONED: LUIS'S SANCTUARY

4

DEDICATION

This book is dedicated to my teachers and supervisors of child psychiatry and psychoanalytic psychotherapy, Mae McMillan, Irv Kraft, Jim Robinson, Hal Boylston, Bill Moore, and Jim Heald. They helped me listen to children and adolescents share their own world, and not superimpose my own.

1—A BOY WHO LOVED KNIVES

OF KNIFE AND MEN

Ever since its invention by humans, the knife, like fire, has many domains of action, meaning, and symbolism. Fire can provide warmth, cook food, and provide light in darkness. Fire can also destroy homes and forests, and kill and torture humans. Psychologically, humans can burn with anger, passion and shame.

A knife can be used to cut food, carve wood into elegant art forms and, in the hands of skilled surgeons, save lives. The knife also can be used to threaten, hurt or kill. When people make difficult decisions they "cutoff" some options. A sharp tongue can use words to cut like a knife. Financial budget cuts hurt, but can save a family or national economy. A truth vigorously applied is said to "cut to the quick". Paradoxically, a sharp knife can be safer than a dull one.

POLICE BLOTTER PREAMBLE

July 4th, 1976

The old man with a Marine Corp KBAR protruding from his left chest close to the sternum had a shaggy gray beard. He was a sturdy-boned five-feet-ten, but had not enjoyed adequate meals for quite some time. He had a fixed stare and had been propped up against a fallen hardwood log near a small, now long-cold cooking fire. There were no signs of a struggle. He had died quickly at the hands of a skilled killer with a sharp combat knife. A police patrol along Buffalo Bayou had discovered the body. What drew the attention of investigators, detective Mark Lane and consultant psychiatrist Dr. Tom Tolman, was the fact that the dead old man's heart had been cut out of his chest and cooked over the nearby fire. The feasting killer had even brought paper napkins and plates. An empty cardboard ice cream container was evidence that the murderer had provided desert for his gruesome meal.

As Lane and Tolman stood observing, they heard the constant rushing sounds of traffic on Houston's West Loop. The bustling traffic on nearby Memorial Drive seemed paradoxical and out of place above the quiet muddy stream that run beneath the busy freeway. The Buffalo Bayou was the hidden waterway of the city's shame where many of Houston's nameless homeless endured mosquito filled nights. Like the New York sewer and subway systems, these grim enclaves, in jungle-like bushes under bridges and next to Houston's bayous and freeways, contain people down on their luck, or forever without it, who chose to be self-appointed iconoclastic human vermin rather than seeking the rejected shelters of misperceived charity. The Houston police make occasional sweeps to break-up what they call the "Bayou City Hobo Camps."

*STOP! The author now makes the following unusual request:

Dear Reader,

Please completely forget the above account of a knife murder. The events described above, never happened! Continue reading to discover how the events above, came never to exist.

Screech!! On Metal: The Wilson Family Music
SCREEEEEEEEEEEEEEECH!

ROBBIE WILSON

The long, endless seeming …SCREECH! Sharpening is accompanied by showers of shiny metal sparks like fireworks flying off the Carborundum grinding wheel at Jack and Jake's Sharpening shop. Now, a welcome soothing silence arrives like a cold drink on a scorching hot summer day.

Robbie Wilson sat in his bedroom staring at his math book. The numbers danced and jumped around on the page. The subtraction stuff was always harder than the addition. Robbie liked things to be added, not taken away. Robbie wished he were with Dad and Uncle Jake out in their backyard shop right now—not in his bedroom, trying to do math homework.

The screech noise used to bug him. When he told his dad, it hurt his ears, his Dad laughed and said, "Robbie my boy, if there were no screeching, our family would starve and have no clothes to wear." Then, after saying stuff like that Dad would laugh.

I love my dad's laugh—it has a music in it. He and Uncle Jake work all day together in their shop behind our house. The big sign on the shop says, JACK & JAKE-R-SHARPER. *They laugh and joke and have fun at work. I don't think too many parents or grown-ups have fun at work. Dad and uncle Jake use ear plugs most of the time during the screeches. But, no screeches allowed after supper. That's when Dad and Jake do paperwork—stuff like printing bills to send, opening mail, licking stamps, recording checks and filling out deposits slips for the bank. Dad and Uncle Jake don't even know it but when I was younger I used to sneak out at night and watch them work and listen to them talk through the screen windows. I hope that I can work with Dad and Uncle Jake someday. The sign on the shop then will say,* JACK, JAKE & ROB-R-SHARPER.

My mom is more serious than dad. Mom's name is Martha. Mom worries a lot. She worries about my school grades. I don't like school. But, Dad says I must get at least through high school so I can work with him and Jake. They say I must be able to add up all our money. Then they laugh. They love to laugh. I want to laugh a lot someday too.

Mom works for the Houston Sewer department. Solid and Liquid Waste Management Department is the real name. Dad and Jake call it the "Poop and Pee Department." Dad kids Mom that she doesn't smell like she works in the sewer. Mom smiles a little when Dad says stuff like that. I think Mom secretly likes Dad's jokes I think they stink but, I laugh too.

I don't know why I stink at school, besides not liking it. I try to study in my room in the evening, but I keep thinking about Dad and Jake at their office out back. I wish I could be grownup already. I wish there was a special time machine that could make me twenty-one right now, rather than only eleven. Mom tries to help me study, but she isn't very good at teaching math.

Dad would be better at teaching me, but he's busy working. Besides, he teaches me all kinds of good stuff about knives, swords, bayonets, lawnmowers, scythes, sickles, hatchets, axes, saws, chainsaws, tree trimmers, strop razors, hedge trimmers, machetes, sabers, daggers, throwing knives, fencing foils, rapiers, scalpels, switch-blades, fighting knives, pocket knives, Swiss Army knives, Boy Scout knives, carving knives, kitchen knives, and Exacta knives. My favorite knife is a United States Marine KBAR knife. My grandpa Johnnie was a marine. He left the KBAR to me when he died. Marine's use their K Bar in combat, to hack through jungles, to help dig foxholes, and even open cans of beans. Dad and Jake say good knife sharpening takes special skill, care and love. They say it's an art—then they laugh their musical laughs.

See you later. I really got to try to study now...."

JAMES LORD, MD

Jim Lord at six feet tall is slender and well-muscled. His handsome face, reddish blonde hair, and quick smile, resemble Robert Redford. His first year of psychiatry residency had gone well. Working with the hospitalized acutely mentally ill had been a fascinating challenge. Lord remembered the moment he decided he wanted to be a psychiatrist as if it were yesterday.

It was a hot spring day during his second year in college. On the same day that Lord broke his leg sliding into home plate at a baseball game, a huge tackle on the football team broke his femur during, and an all-American quarterback tore up his knee. All three men ended up lying in the same infirmary room ensconced in plaster casts and on pain medications. That evening the big tackle got fearful, anxious and paranoid. He said that the doctor and nurse were poisoning him with the injections. He said he might have to hurt or kill people. As Jim began to talk to their roommate, the quarterback buzzed the nurse and handed her a note about the need for help. The young man listened to Jim. When a doctor, who had been summoned by the nurse, arrived and suggested that the tackle needed to go to a special hospital for more treatment, the tackle at first refused but then changed his mind when Jim agreed to accompany him to the hospital. Jim rode the ambulance with his roommate speaking as soothing and reassuring words as he could muster. After midnight, once the tackle was sedated and resting at the hospital, Jim was taken back to the college infirmary. The quarterback told Jim that he should be a psychiatrist. Jim was surprised but pleased at the all-American's compliment. Jim got serious about his pre-med courses and did well enough to get accepted to medical school. After med school Lord had eagerly plunged into his psychiatric training.

Today however Dr. Lord is tense and anxious. Now in his second year, he is required to evaluate and treat kids. *How the hell do you treat kids with mental problems?* Jim was glad that Dr. Tom Tolman would be his supervisor. Tolman had a good reputation as a professor of psychiatry and psychotherapy. Tolman is married to an ex-nun named Andrea, who is another renowned Houston psychotherapist.

Jim knew he would need good supervision because he has no children or siblings and, frankly, doesn't like noisy snotty-nosed kids in general. *How can I treat or cure children if they didn't need medications for things like depression, hyperactivity or ADHD? How am I supposed to treat kids by merely talking to them?*

Lord's palms were sweaty, his neck tense, but the time had come. Robbie Wilson and his mother sat in the waiting room at the Houston Child Psychiatry Clinic. Robbie hated being there. Martha Wilson, hoped for help. Jim Lord hoped that he could figure out how to help his newest patient. [Note: Tried to give the three of them thoughts as the process begins. You may have entirely different ideas about Jim's feeling now.]

****

To train resident physicians in psychiatry and to promote objective observation and reliable medical record-keeping, university hospitals and clinics require careful and meticulously organized record forms. Some observers could say that medical forms are a domain where hard science does devilish dances with scientism. Others cynically say records are for protection against lawsuits. If the clinician doesn't write it down, the court treats it as if the good thing they did doesn't even exist. This allows mistakes to stand out in relief. One of Lord's medical school teachers said records "allow science and technology to protect helpers master primitive fear, superstition and doubt."

Jim Lord, like most doctors, hated paperwork. But, he gritted his teeth and sat down, like a good boy, to write his report.

EVALUATION FORM: HOUSTON CHILD PSYCHIATRY CLINIC

DENTIFYING INFORMATION:

Name: Robbie Wilson. Male. Eleven years old. Grade five. Accompanied by his mother, Martha Wilson age 42. Occupation: Secretary, City of Houston—Department of Solid and Liquid Waste Management. Father: Jack Wilson age 45. Occupation: Owner, Wilson Knife Sharpening Company ("JACK & JAKE-R-SHARPER"). Father is currently at work.

PRESENTING PROBLEMS:

1) School failure. 2) Sleep problems. 3)Groin-slapping tic. 4) Grunting and laughing while slapping.

HISTORY OF PRESENTING PROBLEM SITUATION:

Robbie's mother says his sleep problems and tics started abruptly the day after his 6th birthday. Robbie doesn't fear school and readily attends, but his teachers report that Robbie daydreams frequently. Though an adequate reader, he seems to resist retaining information and only makes adequate effort at his math assignments. He likes drawing and prefers to draw "Knights of the Round Table," their armor, their swords, and other weapons. Robbie has no friends at school although he gets along okay with school peers. He does not get into fights and, other than his poor grades and daydreaming, his teachers like him. If a teacher asks Robbie to read out loud, he grunts and slaps his groin. The other children laugh when that occurs, as does Robbie. His mother has tried to invite other boys at school to attend sleepovers at the Wilson home, but Robbie rejects the idea.

FAMILY HISTORY:

Robbie's mother described no major mental illness in either side of the family, but the paternal grandfather had bouts of depression and a drinking problem. The grandfather died the day before Robbie's sixth birthday.

DEVELOPMENTAL AND MEDICAL HISTORY:

Martha Wilson had a normal pregnancy, labor and delivery with Robbie. An only child, Robbie was described as normal in his developmental milestones except for delayed speech. His mother said their pediatrician said Robbie had "Aphrasia." The doctor explained that Robbie had the capacity to talk all along, but not on schedule at two years old. Robbie suddenly commenced completely normal age appropriate speech at age five. He had the usual mumps, measles, and chicken pox but no meningitis or severe infections. His hearing has been tested as normal.

Jim was now ready to write up his observations of what psychiatrists call the patient's "mental status." This portion of the report describes the functioning of the brain and mind of a person at one moment in time, much, like a cardiologist, who after examining and listening a patient's the heart, describes the heart size, sounds, murmurs, rubs or other cardiac sounds. The mental status can, of course, like heart sounds, change at the time of a subsequent observation. Changes over time can have great clinical importance as can the mental status exam.

Jim stood up, stretched for a couple of minutes, organized his thoughts, then sat back down at his desk and began to type.

MENTAL STATUS EXAM:

Robbie Wilson is a casually dressed eleven-year-old boy of average height and weight. He has brown hair and eyes. He makes furtive eye contact if directly questioned. He seems distracted by objects in the clinic office or by life in general. *He's like a little absent-minded little professor.* Robbie is alert and well oriented to person, place, day-of-week, month/year—but not the specific date. His memory is good especially for things he has interested in, but it requires patient probing even prodding to elicit distant memories or details of events. Robbie doesn't seem depressed but is moderately anxious. After his mother is dismissed to the waiting room, he is guarded when asked about his family. His speech is soft but once rapport is established, it has normal flow, rate and quality. It took quite some time to build tentative rapport and barely sufficient trust. Robbie is estimated to be above average in intelligence without any obvious disturbance in thought process or content. Now, he is difficult to engage in active areas where insight or symbolic reasoning could be assessed. He can do math at an appropriate fifth-grade level but has significant anxiety as he utilizes math skills. When the examiner asked Robbie to read from a book Robbie suddenly slapped his groin and made a huffing or grunting noise, followed quickly by a nervous laugh and supercilious grin. When asked, "What just happened?" Robbie shrugged his shoulders and grinned anxiously. His smile was warm and paradoxically engaging despite his obvious embarrassment.

PRELIMINARY DIAGNOSES:

1. School failure—Probably psychogenic

2. Groin-slapping tic—probably psychogenic. Rule out Tourette's syndrome.

3. Sleep Disorder—unknown etiology.

TREATMENT PLAN:

1. Twice weekly individual psychotherapy sessions.

2. Parent and family conferences PRN.

Jim Lord's notes in his personal journal:

My report about Robbie Wilson sounds so dry, impersonal, stilted, and detached. I guess as a doctor I must learn an objective clinical style of writing for reports and courts, but to me, it seems wooden, sterile, lifeless. Psychotherapy work with Robbie Wilson is far from lifeless and, for me at least, is filled with emotion. For months and months, I dreaded each Tuesday and Thursday morning from nine till ten. My supervisor Dr. Tom Tolman was supportive but at the same time firm. Robbie simply wouldn't or couldn't seem to talk with me about his thoughts, fears and feelings. I think Tolman's supervisory process was partially therapy for me. Tolman painstakingly helped me establish good communication with Robbie. Once in frustration Tolman said to me, "Jim Lord, relax! You get so up-tight at times that when you fart it would whistle!"

Then after six months of playing checkers, board games, and throwing a ball back and forth for 'rapport-building,' Tolman recommended that I ask Robbie to draw pictures of what he was thinking and feeling. Those pictures were pure magic for Robbie's psychotherapy treatment process.

THE BLURRY, CREEPY, COLD, SMELLY FUZZIES...HELP!

Robbie Wilson has had his usual difficulties falling asleep. He awakens startled and scared.

It's here again! My whole bedroom is blurry. My eyes are fuzzy. That smell. The cold grabby thing is creeping up my leg. Both legs. It starts at my ankles, then moves up my legs toward my privates. Yike! It's so cold! NO! Don't touch my nuts! Not my privates! NO!

Robbie shrieks, "Help! Mama! Mama!"

Martha Wilson awakes with a start and runs quickly to Robbie's room at the end of the downstairs hall. She finds Robbie huddled on his bed cringing and facing the wall. When Martha holds Robbie, she notes his fixed, detached stare at first, but then, his body tension fades as he slowly accepts comforting.

As Robbie's tension eases Martha's concern grows. *It happened again! I must tell Dr. Lord about these spells. Does Robbie have epilepsy? Or just Bad dreams?*

****

Robbie

Dr. Lord is nice. I see him every Tuesday and Thursday. I look forward to seeing him. I like him, and not just because he doesn't give shots. He wants me to talk but no words come out. I know he wants me to say stuff. I don't know where the words he wants are. I like playing checkers and throwing the Nerf ball with him. Dr. Lord has laughter in his eyes. If he laughed, I think it would have music in it. Maybe doctors aren't allowed to laugh. Maybe they get in trouble for laughing like some kids at school do. I hope he can help me sleep better and stop hitting myself in the nuts. I just can't stop doing that. It just happens sometimes. When the other kids laugh at me my face gets real red. Then, my ears burn. I laugh at myself. Kids say crying is for babies. I don't want to cry, ever.

****

Jim Lord smiled at his young patient, "Robbie, at our talks I would like you to draw pictures about what you think and feel. We could do it like a comic book and put words in the bubbles above the superheroes' heads. Is that OK with you?"

Robbie sat silently with his pencil poised. "Sure. What do you want me to draw?"

"Draw what comes to your mind. Stuff you picture in your mind. Your mom told me you are waking up scared sometimes. You yell for her to help."

Jim Lord sat in the silence. *Tolman has helped me to be comfortable with silence. He says the mind sometimes does hard work during silences in psychotherapy. Like a refueling pit stop in a long road race. Sometimes in fear, the mind hides somewhere during a silence, like in a game of hide-and-go-seek. Kids imagine, that you can't be seen, hurt or embarrassed in a safe hiding place. Tolman says the psychotherapist can benefit by exploring his or her own feelings during the silence or about the silence. Jim finally felt comfortable in and OK with silence in his therapy with Robbie.*

Robbie reached out toward his new drawing pad. He drew an oblong egg-shaped object with spikes protruding outward from most of the surfaces. He drew with a remarkably accurate three-dimensional quality.

At a recent supervision session, Tolman cautioned Lord that Robbie should not be interrogated, but would gradually and hopefully begin to put his own words onto the pictures. Tolman said connecting words with feelings, bodily sensations and memories had in and of itself, an inherent therapeutic benefit. But, the therapist best not impose his words on the patient. Even if they accurately fit the feelings, inhibitions, fears or conflicts. The challenge for the child therapist, according to Tolman, is how to entwine rapport-building with the stirring of curiosity. Kids are naturally curious, but they learn too soon that many adults are uncomfortable with children's curiosity. Especially curiosity about sex, silliness, body sounds, harmful aggression, and especially, death.

Finally, Robbie drew stick figure arms and legs on the oval drawn previously. It was perched like a head on top of a short stick neck. "I don't like the fuzzy thing in my dream. It scares me."

"Robbie, are you scared that if you go to sleep you will dream about the scary fuzzy thing?"

"I don't always dream when I sleep—only sometimes."

"Do you know what the fuzzy thing is? You drew arms or legs on it."

Robbie responded, "I can't tell if it is an animal, a person, or what?"

Lord recalled that during his evaluation sessions with Robbie, he had asked the standard child psychiatry animal question—if your family were animals what animals would they be?

Robbie answered, "My mother would be a big fat lady cow. My father and uncle would be two male tigers."

"What about your grandfather?"

Robbie paused, touched his inner thigh but didn't slap his groin, then said, "An old lion, but he's dead." Robbie himself would be a tiger cub.

The time for their session was up. Tolman had helped Jim to be mindful not to open new issues at the very end of a therapy session. Tolman said it was like lancing a boil open without time to sew up the wound and bandage properly. So, Jim Lord said,

"Robbie, next time let's talk more about that fuzzy scary thing. See you next time."

****

At their next session, Robbie seemed distracted. He grabbed the Nerf ball and threw it forcefully at Lord. Robbie laughed and said, "Nice catch Dr. Lord, you must have been a good baseball player. I wish I was a better baseball player. The boys at school always pick me near last, and for the outfield where nobody hits the ball much. Once, in the outfield, my mind was picturing Dad and Uncle Jake at their shop. Right then a ball was hit right at me but it bounced through my legs and all the way to the outfield fence. Everyone was mad at me for letting a home run get past me."

Lord wanted to get back to discussion of the fuzzy scary thing, but recalled Tolman's admonitions about not imposing his own curiosity. Lord chose silence and tossed the ball back to Robbie who caught it deftly.

Lord said, "Nice catch Robbie."

More silence. Robbie began drawing and humming for about ten or fifteen minutes. The tune he sounded like the old song, "When Johnnie comes marching home." Then Robbie suggested they play checkers. They each won one game before the time was up.

As he left Robbie said, "Dr. Lord, I want to take my drawing with me and work on it more before we put it in my folder. See you next time Dr. Smiley."

Robbie laughed and he headed to the door.

Lord smiled at Robbie's sarcasm and chuckled to himself.

****

TEACHERS

It had been another tough day at school for Robbie. When Mrs. Klein had asked him to read from their social studies book, Robbie stood up and tried to be brave. Suddenly, he hit himself in the nuts. Damn it! He just couldn't stop that. It was like a magic Halloween ghost put a spell on his arm and hand. Like usual, the kids laughed and his face got really red. Robbie tried to laugh with them. Mrs. Klein hushed the other kids and asked Larry Jones to read. Robbie imagined he was like Peter Pan in the movie. He could fly away for a while. The only place he could fly now was into his thoughts. Thoughts are safe places sometimes. If he were alone, he would hum his special song called, "When Robbie comes marching home." When he was alive, Grampa Wilson used to hum and sing that song to himself. "When Johnnie comes marching home, hurrah, hurrah." Mom told Robbie once that Grampa had been shot during the war. She said once that was why Grampa drank too much beer sometimes. So, he could forget being shot. Beer also helped Grampa fall asleep.

I like Mrs. Klein. Sometimes I like a school teacher but not many of them. So many teachers just tell you stuff in a bossy way. Good teachers are good smilers. Those good teachers really listen. Their eyes say I like you—I want you to learn. They like to hear your questions, even when they don't know the answer. They smile with you and say things like, "Robbie, let's look that up in a book. Next time during your library period look it up for us. I will too." Good teachers remember to discuss the answer at the next class. That makes a book fun for a while. Like a book reading detective.

I like drawing pictures for Dr. Lord. He keeps my drawings in a special folder with my name on it. I like that I have a special folder. I wish Dr. Lord would laugh sometimes. But, he does seem to like me to share my drawings and we talk about them. I liked it when Dad and Uncle Jake used to like my drawings of knives, swords, axes and bayonets. When I drew other

things like trees, dogs and people they didn't pay good attention to those pictures. I wish Dr.
Lord could meet my Dad and Uncle Jake. I think he would like them like I do. Sometimes, I think
I will draw a picture of Dad, Uncle Jake and me for Dr. Lord. "

****

Jim Lord had begun to look forward to his supervisory sessions with Tom Tolman. This was especially true now that Robbie Wilson's "I think and I feel drawings" had opened whole new world in the therapy. Today at supervision, Lord and Tolman studied Robbie's new drawing of his uncle Jake and his father.

Tolman observed, "Jim, notice in Robbie's drawing he is peering through a window into his father's knife sharpening shop. The stick figures for the two adults are drawn with smiling faces but it looks like they are dueling with two swords, a cutlass and a broad sword."

Lord said, "Robbie told me his father and uncle were good sword fighters and he didn't watch long because he was sneaking out to watch the men in the evening when he was supposed to be in his room doing school work. Robbie said he secretly watched his father and uncle through that same window, even when he was a little kid."

Tolman looked closely at Robbie's picture. "It looks like the swords are aimed or swung at Jake and Jack's genitals! Did Robbie say if they got hurt?

"Robbie said, he heard them joke and laugh about cutting each other in the nuts. Robbie said that he was scared at first. But his dad and Jake laughed and giggled so he didn't stay scared. I asked Robbie if his dad and Jake had done the same sword play when Robbie was little. He couldn't remember. He told me that he didn't sneak out there much back then because he got real scared of the dark. I didn't explore the scene any further because Robbie wanted to draw me lots of pictures of swords and fighting knives."

Tolman talked at length about how children's drawings are at times like dreams or daydreams. The drawings solve, or try to solve and resolve conflicts, negotiate developmental hurdles, answer questions on their mind, overcome fears, and solve sexual mysteries. Finally, Tolman said, "Jim, it's time to invite Robbie's father and his uncle Jake to a session."

Lord agreed, but felt very nervous about such a session. Lord asked Tolman if Robbie should be at the session with his father and uncle. Tolman felt that Robbie should have the choice. At Robbie's age and with his good rapport with Lord, he could handle it.

At Robbie's next session he was fidgety. He tossed the Nerf ball and they played checkers. When Lord asked about inviting Robbie's father and uncle to the next session, Robbie didn't object. In fact, he seemed to relish the prospect.

After their session, Lord asked Mrs. Wilson to invite her husband and Robbie's Uncle Jake to Robbie's next session. Martha Wilson smiled and seemed pleased.

MEN IN THE FAMILY: Jack and Jake Wilson.

Jim Lord tried to prepare himself for the meeting with Robbie Wilson's father and uncle. Lord was tense but eager to meet them. The words of a poem by Dr. Tom Tolman's wife, Andrea, came to mind.

FAMILY

A view of Society's fragile existential glue
Composed of hearts bound with love and hate,

We euphemistically call, 'family values'.
They search my face in their vulnerability.
Fearing my words as if they were scalpels;
Anticipating pain of truths quite unwanted.
They struggle to prevent inevitable change,
Constructing coarse cobwebs of smug smiles.
Guarding their feelings with steel walls
A masquerade of spurious protection is,
Merely composed of each other's strengths.
Family fears forming desperate projections,
Hiding their freedom with trivial talking.
I must take risks with my inner family;
To make an awkward contact with theirs.
Where do credentials come from for this?
An attempted delicate journey together.

Jack and Jake Wilson looked remarkably alike. Jack was two years older than Jake and a couple of inches taller. They presented like two mischievous boys with ready but nervous smiles, and they had a Billy Budd innocence about them. They tousled Robbie's hair as the four of them walked down the hall to Lord's office. Robbie took his usual chair near his drawing table and Jack and Jake sat next to each other on the couch facing Lord. Jim intuitively liked Jack and Jake. Robbie seemed comfortable, even pleased in their presence.

Lord resolved to suspend a final opinion about the brothers Wilson saying, "Thank you both for coming. Tell me about yourselves and your relationships with Robbie."

Jake Wilson spoke first saying, "When Martha said you wanted to meet with us I was glad to come. Doctor, I guess you know that Jack and I work together, and I room at Jack and Martha's house. Our dad Johnnie built the house and our shop. Dad taught us the business which Jack and I have run now for many years. Dad retired early with a heart condition. I'd say we are a close family that works hard. "

Lord asked, "Jake, does your wife live in the house with you?"

Jake gazed off and thought a minute before saying, "I've never married. My high school sweetheart and I were engaged but when she died in a car wreck three month before our wedding, I guess I never got over it."

Jake had grown misty-eyed and Jack patted him on the shoulder supportively, saying, "Doctor, how can we help you to help Robbie with his school problem and that groin slapping thing?"

Robbie grinned, blushed and grabbed his crotch gently without an abrupt slap.

Maybe Robbie shouldn't be here for this? But, I sense I can go for it directly so here goes.

"Jack and Jake, Robbie has kind of been a young detective with you guys. Even when he was little, he would want to be near you. So, he snuck outside to a window at your business building and watched you two through the window. Sometimes you guys apparently were play-acting with swords like you were cutting at each other's nuts. That both scared Robbie and fascinated him. As he has gotten older he knows that you would never hurt each other. But, back when he was little, the scary dark and his young mind may have taken those things wrong."

Jack and Jake looked startled and alarmed. Jack Wilson looked genuinely concerned and said sheepishly but intensely, "Doc we did sometimes have a few beers on Friday nights and would kid around with fake sword or knife play. Shoot Doc, we had no idea Robbie was watching or might be hurt or scared by it."

Robbie grimaced, stared, paying close attention.

Lord said, "It probably did scare Robbie when he was little kid. But he and I will work hard together to help him get his mind caught-up and strong. The fact that you men came today and clearly want to help Robbie is very important and helpful."

The rest of the hour provided further information about family activities and further information about family history. Johnnie Wilson, Robbie's grandfather, was discussed. Jack and Jake cleared idealized their father and were clearly grateful to him as the provider of their occupation and livelihood. They were unclear about Johnnie's combat wounds in WWII, the details about his heart condition, or when he fully retired. They both acknowledged that Johnnie drank too much but said he was always available to consult if they had a business or technical sharpening problem. Jack said that Johnnie was close to Robbie and would frequently baby sit with Robbie on Friday nights so Jack and Martha could go out to dinner and a movie. Robbie always looked forward to grandpa's ice cream treat.

Lord noticed that during the last twenty minutes of the session Robbie seemed less attentive, pensive and almost drowsy at times.

****

Robbie's mother called to cancel his next session with Jim. Martha Wilson said that Robbie had stomach flu, had missed school, that his sleep problems had worsened, and that he had one of his nighttime scary spells.

At the next session Robbie appeared subdued, even sullen. They sat in silence for a while until Robbie said, "I don't want to come here anymore."

"Robbie, did something come up after our meeting with your dad and Uncle Jake?"

Robbie looked down toward the floor, "Nope. We just went out for a burger and fries."

"Robbie, your mom told me that you had a stomach ache, your sleep problem is worse, and you had another scary dream thing."

Robbie looked sad as he said, "Yeah and I knew if I went to school I'd probably hit my nuts even more."

Robbie tossed the Nerf ball up and down for a while. When Lord invited him to draw a picture of his feelings Robbie drew a picture of his favorite U.S. Marine K Bar knife with some blood dripping off it. Then, he scribbled over his drawing and said, "I got to go pee and then have my mom take me home so I can take my stomach medicine."

Lord remembered Tolman saying that interruptions to pee during child therapy indicated increased inner tension, sometimes a symbolic equivalent of weeping or repressed rage.

Robbie quickly went over to the door of Lord's office to leave. Jim said, "I'll see you next time." But Robbie shook his head no.

The next day Martha Wilson called Jim Lord to report that Robbie reluctantly went to school but, only when his dad drove him. The sleep problems and nightmares continued. Lord emphasized how important it was for Martha or Jack Wilson to bring Robbie to his next session.

****

TO STAB OR NOT TO STAB.

Robbie stared at the Buck Ranger Skinner knife his dad had given him last Christmas. It was his second favorite to his U.S. Marine K Bar that his grandpa Johnnie used when he was a marine. Grandpa Johnnie left him the K Bar in his will when he died.

Robbie loved the Ranger Skinner knife's short sharp sturdy steel three and one-eighth inch blade. The smooth Dymondwood handle fit just right in his hand. The Ranger Skinner looked cool in its dark brown sheath. When he was hiking in Bear Creek Park sometimes with his dad, Robbie felt strong and safe. Robbie stared at the blade. I thought I liked Dr. Lord. But now I wish I could stick him with this knife. Then he would hurt like I did when he got me to tattle on Dad and Uncle Jake. I am a rat fink for telling on them. I am pissed at Dr. Lord. Mom and Dad say I got to see Dr. Lord today. I'll only go because Dad is taking me. My stomach hurts bad now.

****

Before Robbie and his dad left for the appointment with Dr. Lord, Robbie slid the Ranger Skinner knife and its Sheath into the side button-down pocket of his Camo pants. I don't want to talk to Dr. Lord today or draw stupid pictures. Dad says I got to see him. Crap, my stomach hurts. I wish Dr. Lord would lose sleep and hit his nuts sometimes.

Robbie smiled a little grimly when his dad called him to go to his appointment.

****

Jim Lord was glad to see Robbie and his dad in the waiting room. As their session began Robbie seemed distracted, restless, and distant. When asked to draw pictures about his feelings, Robbie refused. He fiddled with the buttoned pocket of his Camo pants.

"Robbie, you haven't worn those pants before. They have cool pockets to keep stuff. What do you have in the pocket today?"

Robbie frowned, blushed and rubbed his stomach. With his other hand, Robbie unbuttoned the pocket flap and pulled out the Ranger Skinner knife in its sheath. "I thought about sticking you with this knife when you made me rat on Dad and Uncle Jake. I could sure draw a bloody picture of my thoughts about you."

"It's good you brought up your angry thoughts about me. But, it was helpful that your dad, Jake, you and me all could talk about what got you scared as a younger kid. Your dad and Uncle Jake don't see you as rat finking on them. As you grow older now you don't have to lose sleep or get scared about stuff. You can picture fears in your mind and find words for them. Then you can find out what to do about them without anyone getting hurt. Tell me about your knife."

Robbie was quiet for a while. He gripped the knife tightly. He looked doubtful at first but gradually grew more relaxed as he talked about the Ranger Skinner Knife. With some enthusiasm, he talked about what the cowboys used it for on the cattle ranches. Robbie also drew a picture of the throwing knife that his dad taught him to throw at dead tree stumps at Bear Creek Park. After letting Jim Lord admire it, Robbie put the Ranger Skinner knife in its sheath back in his pocket. Before Robbie left the session, he handed the picture of the throwing knife to Jim to put in his special clinic folder.

****

At their supervision session Tom Tolman listened carefully and then asked Jim questions about Robbie's contemplated attack and Jim's reaction to the incident.

"Jim, what was Robbie telling you?"

Jim responded, "I have no idea beside how important his dad and uncle are to him. Also, how protective he is towards them. I thought therapy had been going well but his thinking about knifing me got scary. Does he have thoughts of castrating me?

Tolman said, "You may not agree but I think Robbie's therapy has made real progress. Your tuning into your intuitions shows you are making good progress as a therapist. Even if you don't feel like it Jim, I can see it. Robbie's response to your clarifying intervention tells me that the therapy is on track.

"About your question about castration, I assume the picture he made of the throwing knife had no blood on it. There may be someone else in Robbie's unconscious mind that knifing is intended for, but it isn't you. By the way, I think you should see Robbie's dad, or dad and mom after one of Robbie's sessions each week for a while. Some family secrets might be emerging and hopefully the Wilson family is able do the work to resolve them."

Jim checked the throwing knife picture. The red crayon had not been used on the knife picture. He felt good about the session with Tolman. He knew that Tolman would not make idle complements about his work unless they were authentic.

Martha Wilson called the next day and left a message indicating that Robbie had a bad dream and had missed school again. Robbie had a stomachache. Jim thought, "Like Tolman often says, "One step forward two steps back."

****

Robbie was more relaxed at his next session. He played some checkers with Jim but spoke about how much he had begun to hate school. After the session, Jim Lord met with Robbie's mother.

Martha Wilson was dressed neatly in a conservative looking gray pants suit. She had her gray hair in a ponytail. She had an attractive figure but her tense clenched jaw and hands matched her furrowed brow. She described Robbie's fearful awakening from his nightmare.

Lord asked, "Ms. Wilson, tell me more about Robbie and his sleep patterns."

"Dr. Lord, Robbie's nightmares and sleep have always been a problem. But, they are worse recently. I have noticed they are more likely to occur on Friday nights or rarely on Sunday night. Jack and I like to go out for dinner and a movie on Friday nights. The teenage girls in the neighborhood used to baby sit when Robbie was little but Robbie never wanted a boy baby sitter. Jake sometimes stays with Robbie when we are out which Robbie likes. His grandpa Johnnie was Robbie's favorite baby sitter because he always had ice cream for them to enjoy."

"Do you remember how Robbie reacted when your father-in-law died?"

Mrs. Wilson told Lord that Robbie's grandpa Johnnie Wilson died when Robbie was five. His grandpa had been babysitting Robbie that night. Jack and Martha Wilson returned home after a movie to find Johnnie lying dead on his bed and Robbie was sitting frozen-like on a chair near his dead grandfather. They all were shocked.

"Had Johnnie been drinking that evening?"

Mrs. Wilson looked tense but responded quickly, "Johnnie drank too much beer. He had been drinking even more the months before he died. His doctor had cautioned him about his beer belly and weight gain. We thought Johnnie only drank after Robbie was asleep or after we got home after the movie. Many other nights I heard Johnnie pop beers late at night in the kitchen.

She went on tearfully, "The night we found Johnnie dead, there was noticeable beer smell around his bed where he had been reading to Robbie about Marine Corp history. We sometimes found both Robbie and Johnnie asleep when we got home from a late movie but I don't remember beer smell like that before that night."

At their next supervisory meeting, Tom agreed with Jim that he and Robbie needed to talk about the night Johnnie died.

Jim awaited Robbie's next session with anxiety. He felt tension in his neck and, like Robbie, Jim had a queasy stomach before Robbie entered his office. Robbie seemed more relaxed than Lord as the session started.

"Robbie, we need to talk or draw pictures of the night your grandpa Johnnie died. Your mom talked to me about that night when they found Johnnie dead and you sitting nearby his bed. He had been reading to you about Marines."

Robbie grabbed his stomach and slapped his groin with a low groaning sound. Robbie started to move toward the door. Jim said, "Don't leave. Tell me or draw me a picture of what happened."

Robbie grew tight-lipped and began to draw rapidly on paper. He drew a crude sketch of Johnnie's bed with a book beside Johnnie on the bed and Robbie standing near the bed and punching Johnnie in the chest. Robbie then sat dazed staring at Dr. Lord.

"Robbie, did your grandpa touch you?"

Robbie drew a quick sketch of the fuzzy round thing he had drawn for Lord before and said, "I liked the stories about the Marines but Grandpa was crying and talking funny about his buddies dying. He had that stinky smell of beer and he was hugging me and feeling my legs and moving up toward my nuts. I punched him hard in his chest and got out of his bed. Grandpa got a scared look on his face and couldn't breathe. I killed Grandpa! I know I did!" Robbie slumped in his chair and scratched across his pictures with a pencil.

"Robbie. You did not kill your grandpa. The doctors knew he had a heart problem and he died from a heart attack. Not your punch."

Robbie started to cry saying in a bitter tone, "How do you know Dr. Lord?"

"Because I'm a doctor that knows about heart attacks as well as problems with fears and feelings. I can find Johnnie's medical records for us to read and even have you and I talk to his doctor to prove that he died from a heart attack and not your punch."

"You would do that with me, Dr. Lord?"

"Yes, I would and I also want you to know that Johnnie's touching of you was wrong. That was his problem, not yours! It was good for you to punch him to make him stop. I think we will find out together that Johnnie's touching your legs and nuts makes you have sleep problems and is the reason why you're hitting yourself in the nuts."

There was a long silence during which Robbie slowly stopped crying and Jim took some deep breaths until his neck tension and queasy stomach disappeared. Robbie put his drawings in his folder and handed it to Jim.

"Robbie, I'll see you next time."

Robbie had no comment and joined his father in the waiting room.

****

Several follow-up sessions with Martha, Jack, and Jake Wilson were poignantly defined. At first all three adults were stunned, disbelieving, and then tearful. Then, with Jim's support, they began to talk about the Johnnie Wilson they had loved, put on a pedestal, and been intimidated by. Jack and Martha agreed to obtain Johnnie's medical and autopsy record and ask Johnnie's doctor if he would explain Johnnie's death to Robbie in person if Jim Lord felt it was necessary.

At their final session, Jake Wilson surprised Martha and Jack by reporting that he had confronted Johnnie about drinking beer around Robbie. Johnnie denied drinking when he and Robbie were alone together, and Johnnie's behavior had improved for a while. Jake also described a fuzzy scruffy-looking beard that Johnnie had sported the last few months of his life. Johnnie told Jake that during bitter battles with the Japanese he and his marine buddies had all grown beards. Neither Jake, nor Jack, nor Martha had any inkling that Johnnie might have fondled Robbie.

****

Talking with Johnnie's doctor, Cliff Peterson, was helpful. Robbie asked Peterson directly if he had caused his Grandpa's death. Peterson impressed Lord by treating Robbie's question seriously, clearly and kindly. Robbie appeared satisfied with the answers.

Robbie's subsequent sessions with Jim Lord were lively with fun Nerf ball throwing. Robbie drew many pictures for his folder. He drew several pictures of the "smelly, fuzzy bad guy." The bad guy got chased away by Robbie holding his Ranger Skinner knife. After these active sessions, Robbie ceased having nightmares. He no longer feared embarrassing groin-slapping episodes, because they had completely ceased. Lord, Robbie's teacher and especially Robbie were pleased.

Jim spent a final supervisory session with Tom Tolman talking about how he was going to miss Robbie. He thanked Tolman for his help and told him that he had decided to go into child psychiatry, specializing in child psychotherapy.

After Jim left his office, Tom leaned back in his chair and enjoyed the feeling that came from being a teacher of psychotherapy and passing on his knowledge and experience to a talented young doctor like Jim

In the final months of his psychotherapy, Robbie talked about how much he was enjoying school. He was looking forward to the baseball season because his dad had been practicing with Robbie and his friends. At his final session, Robbie gave Lord an early Christmas gift—a Swiss Army knife. Robbie promised that he, Jake, or his dad would be glad to sharpen it anytime it needed it.

LESSONS LEARNED FROM ROBBIE WILSON

Jim Lord's Notes:

Work with Robbie taught me that family resilience sometimes provides a valuable synchrony in support of a child's cure in psychotherapy. Family history of secrets, abuse and conflicts comes to life therapeutically when family members have the courage to confront issues and deal with them in treatment.

In addition, the use of a child's drawings or other art modalities can be very helpful during the therapy process.

2—A BOY WHO WATCHED HIS FATHER MURDERED

> The tissue of society can be destroyed where violators of human rights enjoy
> impunity; are not prosecuted; trauma continues without ways to mourn the losses;
> there is no way to recognize the suffering of victims; and no moral or economic
> reparation. —Elizabeth Rohr

Dr. Juan Gomez was during presenting a patient's case history to Dr. Tom Tolman, the unit staff,

and his psychiatry resident colleagues when he abruptly burst into tears. Gomez excused himself

from the conference room and headed down the hall to his office. Tom Tolman followed and

discovered Juan sitting at his desk sobbing. Tolman regarded Gomez as a kind and good soul. As

Juan used Kleenex, Tolman sat quietly. Gomez was respected, even loved by hospital staff and

his colleagues. The head nurse came to the door of Gomez's office asking if anything was

needed. Tolman told her things were okay and asked her to call his private office and have his

secretary cancel all his afternoon patients. Then Tolman sat ready to listen.

THE VETERANS ADMINISTRATION HOSPITAL

Tom Tolman enjoyed his psychiatric work at Houston's Veterans Administration Hospital. Such

positive feelings about the VA were unusual considering recent national scandals about massive

problems in the VA healthcare system. As a medical student and a resident doctor of psychiatry

Tolman had had good teachers and interesting patients with which to work. Many of his

colleagues at the time called it the VAAAAH and disrespectfully called the frequent alcoholic

emergency room patients, "VA trolls."

Now as a senior faculty psychiatrist at the Houston medical schools, Tolman enjoyed part-time work teaching residents in psychiatry. Tolman worked mornings at the VA and afternoons in his private practice office. The regular paycheck and health insurance coverage as a VA doctor was valuable, but in addition, Tolman felt a loyalty to the VA.

Not only did he have good memories of his student days at the VA, but he felt especially loyal to the Vietnam War veterans who he had treated during his two years of U.S. Navy duty. He respected his chief on the locked psychiatry unit because the chief insisted that both he and Tolman each carry the same patient load as the resident doctors. Each Tuesday and Thursday Tolman met with the several residents on the unit as a group. He also spent an hour each week with the each of residents in individual supervision about their cases. His door was always open for a resident who had a difficult patient situation to discuss.

DOMAINS OF TEARS

After an unnecessary apology by Gomez was brushed aside by Tolman, Juan began to talk, "I embarrassed myself with you, the staff, my colleagues and, most of all, my patient, Mr. Hernandez. I was taking Hernandez's history when I suddenly lost it, burst into tears and blacked out about the details of what we were talking about. I told Mr. Hernandez that I wasn't feeling well and that I would finish our talk later that day. Late that afternoon I talked with Hernandez and again burst into tears and had to stop again. Am I going psychotic Dr. Tolman? I don't feel depressed and I like my work and training."

"Juan, do you take notes or record your initial patient histories and physicals?"

Gomez reached into the desk drawer for a folder. "I always take minimal shorthand notes during the interview and then dictate the full text later. I like to look at the patient to establish rapport and observe his behavior."

"Maybe if you look through your notes you will recall the details of the Hernandez interview. First, close your eyes and take some deep relaxing breaths. We have plenty of time."

Gomez leaned back in his chair and closed his eyes. After a few minutes he opened his eyes, looked at his notes and said, "My notes indicate Tony Hernandez was articulate and a good historian. He told me that he had felt sad, depressed and empty since right after he got out of the Navy. I asked him if he missed the Navy and he said, 'Yes.' But he wanted to continue to go to sea and work on his dad's fleet of fishing boats out of Galveston. According to my notes, his dad had been in the Navy too. I asked him to tell me about his father. Hernandez told me that he and his dad were very close and they partied the afternoon and evening after Tony got home after his discharge from the Navy. My notes stop there. The paper is stained with my tear drops. I can't picture any more from there. "

Juan took more deep breaths, tried, but couldn't recall any more events. He had stopped crying and looked bewildered, perplexed, and obviously worried. Tom told Juan that they could use hypnosis but first he suggested that he and Juan interview Tony Hernandez together. Maybe important information would emerge. Juan agreed with some trepidation and the interview with Tony Hernandez was arranged the next morning at Juan's hospital office.

Juan paid close attention as Tolman began the interview with Tony Hernandez. At Tolman's request, Hernandez described how he and his dad had partied at Randy's bar till shortly before midnight. "We were both drunk but my friend Earl who was with us had agreed to be the designated driver. Earlier in the evening a former employee of Dad's came into the bar. When he saw Dad, he scowled, sneered and quickly left. Dad told me that the man was pissed about being fired the previous year. Later, as the three of us walked towards the car, the former employee jumped out from behind another car and shot Dad in the chest. Blood covered Dad's fancy shirt. He died quickly as I knelt by him on the ground."

Juan stood up, grabbed his chest, and left the office.

Tolman reassured the patient that he and Gomez would help him with his grief and depression but it would take time. The bewildered and anxious Tony Hernandez agreed to a meeting with Tolman at the end of the afternoon.

FINDING THE WORDS TO HEAL

Tolman quickly found Juan sobbing softly in the chair next to Tolman's desk. Tolman sat in his chair prepared to listen. Juan began to talk quietly looking like a person struggling to emerge from a trance, "I loved my daddy. I still see his warm smile. I feel his gentle hug. I smell his Old Spice after-shave lotion. I loved to take walks with Papa downtown in Zona Viva. Those people in Papa's district smiled and greeted the councilman they elected again and again. They loved him and he loved them. Daddy loved them like he loved our family and me.

"Today, like every day in the time before the election Papa walked out on the streets of Zona Viva early in the morning. Mamma smiled her loving sunshine smile at Papa as we left the house. All Guatemala City soon would vote for leaders of our city. Papa knows they will vote for him, but regardless, he loves his people and the campaign trail.

"Since I have no school today I am excited to be asked to walk with him. It is my number eleven birthday and I know Papa will get me a gift today. My little brothers and sisters wish they could go campaigning with Papa like me. The shopkeepers are opening their shops and Papa likes to sip coffee with them. He listens to their problems and ideas. I can't wait for us to reach the candy store. The owner senor Alvarez will give me the candy I choose.

I and Papa turn the corner just before the candy shop. BAM! A man with a mask jumped from the alley and shot Papa. Papa falls. He has blood all over the front of his fancy white shirt. His face is getting very pale very fast. Papa cries out 'Help!' He cries in pain. Papa grabs my hand and says he loves me. He says I must go home quickly to Mamma. I don't want to leave Papa. Mr. Alvarez has called the police and ambulance. He holds a big towel on Papa's chest and tells me to go get Mamma. I run as fast as I can. When I get home, Mamma is crying and our neighbor friend is holding Mamma in her arms. I feel numb. My brothers and sisters stand still and stare at Mamma, who can't stop crying. Our telephone is lying on the floor near Mamma. I can't get out of my numbness. I try to cry but no tears come out of me. My uncle Alberto has come and he holds me and hugs my brothers and sisters too. He has tears streaming down his face. I feel my cheeks but there are no tears. My chest and head aches. My stomach feels bad."

Juan Gomez vomits in Tom Tolman's wastebasket. He begins to cry and sob. Many tissues later, Juan begins to talk to Tom saying, "Now I can see it like it was yesterday. My God! Gomez & Hernandez, Tony & Juan and dead daddies. The black-out blank in my mind is clearing slowly. That must be the reason I had to get away from my talk with Tony Hernandez. Toni's tragic loss merged with mine. Now I am seeing what I had pushed completely out of my mind

Tolman listened. Gomez continued, "Our priest had helped to comfort Mamma, me and my siblings. Uncle Alberto was great. But Mamma was depressed for a long time and our family struggled with finances. My uncle Alberto was part of the U.S. backed prodemocracy government as a soldier. My mother and young siblings were safe with Alberto and his family. The leftist rebels, one of whom likely assassinated my father, were still fighting in a bloody civil war until 1996. I had been very good in school so I was able to get a scholarship to a prep school in Florida and later a scholarship to University of Miami. My med school psychiatry teachers recommended me for a residency at Baylor and that's how I got into this psychiatry residency. I send money to help my mother and two siblings who are now in school.

"What can I do Dr. Tolman? I feel like I'm failing."

Tolman thought for a minute as Juan stared at him anxiously. "Juan, you just began the healing process for yourself moments ago. That's where I think both you and Tony Hernandez begin the grieving and healing. If you can, you need to meet with Tony today and finish taking his history. It will be tough, but on the other hand, I think your own grief process will help you assist Tony to talk through his own grief. That talking cure will add to the antidepressant meds you offer him. I will also refer you to a good psychotherapist to help you continue your own resolution of your grief. I will support you here as you work with Tony Hernandez. I think you are strong enough to do it. What are your thoughts about that idea?"

Juan sat and thought for several minutes. He of course was very anxious about another interview with Hernandez.

"Juan, you know the Texas analogy about the importance of getting right back up on a horse that had thrown you. In the long run, your own grief-work can benefit your inner life and your personal relationships. It can also inform your work with Tony Hernandez and your development as a psychiatrist."

Juan spent an hour beginning his own journey into the process of delayed and unresolved grief-work by further discussion with Tom. He spoke emotionally in more detail and more neutrally about his beloved father.

"Do I tell Tony about my own grief?

Tolman said, "Ultimately that is your choice Juan. But remember that Tony's therapy is the primary issue. What is best for him and his treatment holds priority. Keep your own therapy primarily in the process with your own therapist. If necessary, you could share with Tony that your loss of an important family member caused you to feel strongly when he talked about his loss. It necessitated your interrupting your sessions with him temporarily. But, now you can proceed with confidence that you can help Toni's treatment opportunity to go forward."

Juan took down the names of a woman and a man who Tolman recommended as psychiatrist/psychotherapists whom Juan could call for consultation about his personal psychotherapy. Tolman urged Juan to interview the psychiatrist psychotherapists carefully before beginning his psychotherapy treatment. Juan was surprised but pleased about the freedom to carefully select his own therapist.

Tom was doing paper work late that afternoon when Tony stopped by his office to talk briefly about his interview with Hernandez. Tony described feeling emotionally drained but also relieved that the interview went successfully.

Tom enjoyed teaching and supervising Juan Gomez during the rest of his six-month rotation at the VA hospital. Tom was pleased to watch and hear positive things about Juan's excellent work as a psychiatric resident. Such experiences made the teaching of *The Impossible Profession* worth it.

LESSONS LEARNED FROM JUAN GOMEZ

Tom Tolman's notes:

It is of inestimable value for a psychiatrist, psychologist, psychiatric social worker or psychiatric nurse to have a personal experience in psychotherapy. A personal therapy experience allows the professional to avoid be blinded by their own psychological pain. It also allows the professional to empathize and be more comfortable in helping their patient confront their pain and conflict. Many or most of us in the mental health field have had some significant enough personal pain or conflicts that leads us to work in our field. Such a training psychotherapy is a helpful personal and professional investment.

3—A BOY WHO DIDN'T TALK FOR 40 YEARS

Tom Tolman MD returned to his office at the end of a long day of teaching and committee meetings at the Texas Medical Center. He looked through the stack of phone messages his secretary had left on his desk. One of the constant challenges of the practice of clinical psychiatry and psychotherapy is the triage screening of phone messages. There could literally be dire consequences of an unreturned or postponed phone call. Most psychotherapists have on occasion imagined the guilt and shame they would feel and being ostracized by colleagues and patients if a patient or client called desperate for help and they were unavailable or inattentive. Beyond the fear of malpractice suits, the dose of soul-sadness surrounding a missed opportunity to prevent a suicide or homicide would be huge.

Of the fifteen phone messages, one arresting messages simply stated, "I finally want to talk to you after 40 years. Patrick."

Tolman returned several urgent calls then called Patrick back.

"Hello Patrick, this is Dr. Tolman returning your call. What can I help you with?

"My son Alex has nervous mutism, just like I did when I saw you 40 years ago. Alex is five and he won't talk to me. He won't talk to his preschool teacher, or any other authority figures like a coach, policeman, or our mailman, but he talks easily to my wife and his younger sister. I know you helped me to start talking 40 years ago, so I want your advice."

Tolman knew that Patrick had a successful business, a contented marriage, and four children—two sons older than Alex and Alex's younger sister. Tolman recommended a child psychiatrist close to Patrick's home. Tom told Patrick to let him know if any problems occurred with the referral and to keep in touch about Alex. Patrick expressed gratitude and suggested they talk face-to-face if Tolman visited Patrick's area.

Tom thought---*Wow! It seems like yesterday when I saw Patrick in therapy. Can't believe it was 40 years ago. It wasn't talking therapy of course, because Patrick never said a word to me for the year or more I saw him. I was in my first year of medical school and was looking for a summer elective. I knew I wanted to seriously consider psychiatry as a career. Dr. Alan Croft was offering a summer elective in child psychiatry so I applied. I had heard that Dr. Croft. took a real interest in students and gave them as much responsibility as possible and provided good teaching and supervision. On one hand, I didn't see myself becoming a child psychiatrist, but on the other the chance to work with a man of Dr. Croft's caliber was a real draw.*

Croft and I met with Patrick, his mother and father. I couldn't believe it when Croft made the surprising recommendation to Patrick's parents that I have dinner with Patrick and his family. What? It sounded a bit weird. Croft later explained that a home visit and a school visit, or at least conference with the teacher, was very important so that I could observe Patrick in the real day-to-day world in which he lived. With considerable preliminary curiosity and anxiety, I had dinner with Patrick and his family. I got to their house in Clear Lake about 4 PM so Patrick could show me his room, toys and anything else he cared to show me.

Patrick's mother graciously greeted me and called Patrick and his siblings so she could introduce me. The kids were clearly curious and they chattered with each other in lively fashion. Patrick seemed eager to see me and show me his room. Patrick seemed to experience superior status in the sibling ship via my presence. That surprised me because some clinicians could fear that Patrick might feel stigmatized.

Patrick of course said nothing but at my suggestion drew a picture of himself and his family. When asked the standard questions about what animal would he and his family members be, he drew a cow for his mother, a calf for his younger sister, a lion for his father and lion cubs for his brothers. Patrick was a tiger. Patrick showed me his toy cars, cowboy figurines and his drawing board. He drew a picture of his teacher and his school. When asked whether he liked his teacher he drew a stick figure with a big smile. [Note: a quick reference here such as the two words I added to tie this into the more detailed dinner info in the next paragraph] After dinner,

Patrick showed me the family recreation room and we tossed some rubber horseshoes until I indicated I had to leave. When I told Patrick, I would see him at our appointment the following week he smiled and drew a smiling tiger face.

I reported my observations to Croft who agreed when I said that Patrick had a loving, loyal family. I had noted that Patrick's dad, a PhD with an important role in the NASA space flight program, came in late for dinner and seemed harried and somewhat preoccupied. He tried to speak with Patrick during dinner but Patrick couldn't be drawn into the table conversation. Patrick clearly was listening, grinning and very involved despite his wordlessness.

When we next met, I was pleased that Croft felt my observations were important and supported our preliminary diagnosis that Patrick was not psychotic, considerably above average in intelligence, and his selective mutism was most likely due to social phobia. The selective mute behavior might look on the surface as stubborn defiance but really reflected a mild neurotic way of controlling his anxiety and drawing attention to his needs. My discussions with Croft bolstered my confidence that I as a mere senior medical student was on track with the treatment.

Croft met a final time with Patrick's parents. He told them that I would be Patrick's therapist and that he would meet with them for some couple's therapy sessions and one more time at the end of the summer with Patrick present. Then Croft made an unusual and striking recommendation. He requested that Patrick write me a letter each Christmas that would contain his school picture and a note from him about what he was doing in school and after school. Croft recommended that Patrick and his dad enter karate classes together and that his dad not miss any classes. I saw Patrick twice a week for play therapy sessions without putting any pressure on him to speak. An art therapist named Karen and I co-led an art therapy group that included

Patrick and two of Croft's other patients with selective mutism—Carol, who was six, and Tim, who was five. Patrick's parents readily agreed so I began to see Patrick twice a week. As a first-year medical student, I felt honored, pleased but anxious.

The therapy process was fascinating. Patrick and I played checkers, board games, miniature golf and tossed a ball. On rare occasions, I couldn't resist saying to Patrick that it was okay for him to talk. At such occasions, Patrick smiled and wrote me a brief note or drew me a picture with stick figures of the two of us with our initials under the pictures—his face had no mouth but mine did. He enjoyed showing me his schoolwork and drew pictures of his teacher, classmates and the schoolyard activities. He enjoyed getting me to guess what his pictures were about. If I couldn't guess he would grin and draw additional clarifying pictures. Later in the first year he would write long notes about questions I would ask. The notes and pictures reflected his happiness when he and his dad did things together. In the pictures, Patrick drew of the two of them, they both had smiles on their faces.

My first meeting with Patrick's teacher was very interesting. She had to be reassured that she didn't have to push Patrick to talk and that it was important not to take it personally when Patrick didn't talk to her. By my second meeting a month later with Patrick's teacher, he had begun speaking to her. During a therapy session, I had casually mentioned to Patrick that if he talked to his teacher class would be more fun. Croft felt that was an important intervention. I wasn't as sure. I recall feeling somewhat jealous about Patrick talking to his teacher and not me. But, glad that Patrick was making progress.

Croft kept asking if I was angry at Patrick for not talking. I said no, that I really liked being with Patrick. I had no children at the time and enjoyed our walks together, game playing and Patrick's sense of humor which shone through his drawings and occasional pantomime

performances. When I asked him a direct question that begged an answer, Patrick would put his

index finger over his mouth and laugh. I thought it might mean we had a special secret. Or,

Patrick might fear that if he talked I might declare him cured, and we would no longer meet.

The art therapy play- group sessions Karen and I held were intriguing. After the second

of the four sessions, Carol began to talk freely with Karen and me. Carol aggressively talked to

Patrick and Tim but they stayed silently no matter how verbally active she became. All three

were speaking to Karen by our final session, but neither Tim or Patrick would not talk to me.

They smiled and showed me their art work, but never spoke.

The Karate classes that Tim and his dad and Patrick and his dad were attending were

clearly helping. Soon both Tim and Patrick began speaking to their dads and coaches at school.

I told Croft that Patrick's silence with me seemed to represent a spoken wordless bond that

helped things open with their dads. Croft complimented my idea and my patience. Croft

suggested that if Patrick spoke to me it might interfere with progress relating to his dad.

After about a year-and-a-half of weekly meetings with Patrick, he was doing extremely

well but did not say a word to me even as he hugged me goodbye. The hug said volumes about

the non-verbal therapeutic context of my relationship with Patrick.

Every year for the next forty years, with a few gaps during my moves or changes of

residence and office, Patrick sent me a Christmas card with pictures and written reports of his

progress at school. As Patrick grew into adulthood he wrote to me each Christmas with pictures

of his own family and information about his career, activities and life phase events. In recent years, Patrick and I have corresponded about political and cultural issues in which we share a common interest. Patrick writes eloquently and elegantly about politics.

Our relationship I think has been a remarkable and rewarding relationship without use of vocalization. Patrick's tenacity, intelligence and resilience has been a privilege for me to experience.

LESSONS LEARNED FROM PATRICK

Tom Tolman's notes:

Therapy work with Patrick taught me that while words have great importance, a therapeutic relationship involves important non-verbal aspects. The mentor supervisor Dr. Alan Croft helped establish trust between me, Patrick and his parents. Croft also established safe boundary for the psychotherapy by asking Patrick's parents to invite me to their home for dinner. The value of home visits and teacher conferences during some children's therapy was established in Patrick's situation.

4—A BOY NAMED TOMMY AND HIS MOM & ROADS TO ISIS AND AL QAEDA

Tommy is a dark haired, brown eyed twelve-year old. A serious boy, he rarely smiles, but when he does, his smile accentuates his good looks. Tommy's teacher felt that he was underachieving because of depression. His mother reluctantly brought him for psychiatric evaluation and requested that he receive medication. Dr. Tolman recommended psychotherapy for a while before considering medication for Tommy, Dr. Tolman found Tommy to be bright and articulate during his weekly therapy sessions.

****

TOMMY'S THOUGHTS

I like Dr. Tolman. His eyes smile, but he never laughs at me. He listens to me and likes pictures I draw. Dr. Tolman keeps a special file with my pictures. The file is all for me and no one else but me and him can look at it. I like it that he told my mom that I don't need medicine. Other kids at school get medicines from doctors and it makes them jumpy, sleepy, creepy or goofy.

TOM TOLMAN ONCE WROTE:

Changes occurring in psychotherapy are deceptively quiet, often muted. Psychotherapy involves many emotional experiences: anxiety, fear, fascination, wonder, boredom, humor/laughter, anger, sadness and often pain. However, the more severe and ominous forms of pain, destruction and even a death prevented, go unheralded. They are unnoticed because existentially, like a suicide prevented, they never exist.

Tommy's therapy progressed slowly but steadily. Tommy, an only child, told Dr. Tolman that he missed his dad who had left the home when Tommy was five years old. He had enjoyed fishing and camping with his dad. Tommy's dad continued to see him two weekends every month.

Before his dad moved out, Tommy would overhear his parents have what he described as violent verbal arguments that sometimes involved slapping and hitting. The arguments occurred in his parents' bedroom as they watched movies and TV. Tommy sometimes hoped the fights were only part of the movie. Tommy said his parent's divorce made him feel numb. Sometimes, sad.

During Tommy's seventh session Dr. Tolman explored with Tommy why it was that he never invited friends from school over to his house. Tommy's eyes welled up with tears and he grew silent.

"Why don't you like to bring friends home, Tommy?" Tommy thought for a moment and then said, "It's my mom and her boyfriend. They watch movies and loud TV in their bedroom. They like violent shows like 'Lethal Weapon' or 'Silence of the Lambs'. They smoke marijuana too. If I had friends over, they might get scared. My mom could be in trouble with their parents. At least my mom and Harry don't fight and hit."

Tolman decided that he had to confront Tommy's mom and Harry. He requested their presence at a separate session. Tommy's mom came alone. Vicki was a thirty-seven-year-old strikingly attractive woman with dark brown hair and eyes. She seemed defensive and anxious saying, "What is this about?"

Tolman looked directly at Vicki, "You and Harry's marijuana smoking and the constant diet of violent and sexually explicit movies leads to Tommy feeling lonely, frightened, isolated from his friends, and depressed".

Vicky shot Tolman a disgusted look, "I don't believe that crap! You are a typical anti-pot doc. Tommy has his own TV and he doesn't know about our marijuana because we open the window and keep the door closed."

Tolman said, "Tommy is old enough to realize what pot smells like and the violent and sexual movies you watch both fascinate and frighten him. They stir up memories he has about your fights with his dad in the bedroom when he was little."

She snarled, "That's BS Doc! I need to have a life myself. You won't see Tommy again."

Tolman's voice was measured by calm, "It would be very important for me to see Tommy again, at least to say goodbye. You also need to know that I am reporting you and Harry to Child Protective Services."

Vicki stood, picked up her purse, turned on her heel and stormed from Tolman's office muttering threats about calling her lawyer. Tolman placed a call to CPS.

Several months later, Vicki called to set up an appointment for herself.

"Well, Doc, I guess you thought you never would see me again. After our last talk a CPS worker came to talk to us. I thought you were bluffing. Didn't believe that you would call them. CPS warned us, and I thought a lot about what you said. I told Harry that we couldn't smoke pot around Tommy. Harry got mad and without the pot to mellow us out, sex got worse, and so did the fights. Harry got his own place and now we date only occasionally."

Tommy's mother described how she could not get sexually aroused or have orgasm without the pot and exciting movie scenes of sex and violence.

She said, "Particularly the Mel Gibson or Danny Glover types who are gentle husbands and fathers beneath their gun-prowess, toughness and Adonis bodies. Part of the reason my husband left me seven years ago was because he wasn't interested in what he had labeled, "My real-life pornography of sex, violence and pot."

As a girl, Vicki could recall listening with her sister as her parents used pot, alcohol and had sex. Vicki felt that violence laden movies in her bedroom were safe because no one was hit or hurt. She said this with a seductive smile at Tolman.

"Do you want therapy help with the pot and violent movie addiction?"

Vicki thought for a moment. "Yes. I think I do."

"Vicki, I'm going to refer you to a women psychotherapist, a colleague of mine, who has extensive experience with substance abuse. I also recommend that Tommy's therapy sessions be resumed. And, if your therapist thinks it would be helpful, we can schedule some occasional family sessions. Vicki signed permission for the therapists to confer.

After a brief hospitalization and antidepressant medication, Vicki started to make significant progress

Vicki's therapist told Tolman that the therapy work had been difficult for Vicki. The therapist also said that it had been wise for Tom to refer Vicki to a female therapist because Vicki felt attracted to Tom and had hoped to seduce and break up his marriage.

Vicki worked hard on building credibility and strength in her role as parent. "Parental guidance" became more than a slogan for her. Tommy began to smile more frequently and his teacher was pleased with his improvement at school. Tommy promptly graduated from therapy to return to a now happy boyhood.

Because of his work with Tommy and his mom, Dr. Tolman wrote the following paper.

'THE MEDIA AS MESSAGE': Good News and Bad News for Individual and Cultural Identity

As early as 1964 Marshal McLuhan recognized that in tangible and intangible ways 'The Media is the Message."1* In 1990**, Olsson pointed out that mankind has been pleased by many results of vivid worldwide TV media coverage. Athletes, politicians, educators, poets, symphonies, operas, musicals, ballets and even men on the moon, leap with immediacy into homes all over the world. But, few people anticipated the shocking media power of the bloody results of a terrorist's bomb. Terrorists would pay millions of dollars if they had to pay for media coverage of their kidnappings, skyjackings, assassinations, torturing, and explosions at embassies and streets crowded with civilians. The immediacy of TV and movies form a grandiose mirror and worldwide psychodrama stage for terrorism as a media event.

TV and movie portrayals of violence have concerned parents, pediatricians and child psychiatrists for many years. **The American Academy of Child & Adolescent Psychiatry** (2003***) has pointed out that children watch an average of three to four hours of TV daily.

Adults watch at least that much in addition to both kids and adults watching rented movies. The AACAP points out that the hundreds of research studies on TV violence and kids have found that children may become: (1) "immune" to the horror of violence (2) gradually accept violence to solve problems (3) imitate the violence they observe on TV; and (4) identify with certain characters, victims and/or victimizers.

In my clinical experience, **'Adults'** are also influenced in the same ways [(1) -(4) above] as children. In my opinion, the pornography of movie and TV violence and Hollywood's portrayal of irresponsible sexual behavior leads to ineffective parenting and even increased marital infidelity and probably "Road Rage."

The studies summarized by AACAP also revealed that extensive viewing of violence by children increases aggressiveness, even after the viewing of a single violent program. Children who view violence on TV that is vividly realistic, frequently repeated or unpunished, are likely to imitate what they view. Kids with psychological, behavioral or learning/impulse control problems are more easily influenced towards violent behavior that often occurs many years later and even without overt violence in the household. [Note: Instead of saying "My patient Tommy, I've changed to a "young patient I treated" because original reader of the paper would not have the short story reference to Tommy (which is also a pseudonym so you would have to give "Tommy" another pseudonym here so I thought it might be better to be more generic?] An example of this was a young patient I treated whose situation suggested that he had been constantly depressed and fearful because TV violence was not only enjoyed by his parent, but because his parent had been violent.

The AACAP recommends the following ways for parents to protect children from the impact of TV violence: (1) Parents should pay attention to the programs their children are watching and watch some with them. My patient had left him alone to watch his own TV while his mother enjoyed violent, sexy TV and movies while smoking pot with her boyfriend. (2) Set limits on the amount of time children spend with TV and remove the TV from their rooms. My patient's mother promoted his own TV so she could enjoy hers. (3) Point out to children that the actor in the movie was not actually hurt or killed but that violence in real life would result in pain and or death. (4) Refuse to allow children to see shows known to be violent, and change the channel or turn off the TV when the offensive material comes on with an explanation about what is wrong about the program. Obviously, my patient's mother was unable do any of these things prior to her own psychotherapy. My patient stayed in a fearful cocoon. (5) Disapprove of the violent episodes in front of your children, stressing the belief that such behavior is not the best way to solve the problem. My patient's mother saw the violence as a 'turn-on'. (6) Contact the parents of your child's friends so they can develop similar standards about TV and film violence. My patient feared inviting friends over because of the content of the TV that was shown in his house.

It seems clear to me that 'adults' are also vulnerable to the psychologically adverse effects of TV and movie violence and irresponsible sex. Our American culture seems to be in massive denial of this reality. This is largely because of the profit motive of Hollywood, and our worship of movie star and sports celebrities. Adults who are titillated by the pornography of media sex and violence make totally incompetent parents in terms of primary prevention of violence in future generations.

CONFIRMING DATA FROM THE MEDIA

In the November 3rd, 2003 issue of The New Yorker, George Packer has a poignant article entitled, "Letter from Ivory Coast--- GANSTA WAR: Young fighters take their lead from American pop culture." **** During his descriptions of the deteriorating economic and political situation in Ivory Coast, Packer shares with us descriptions of some of the young adults he got to know. Packer introduces us to Cool B and his friends in the group Cool B leads. Packer describes how these young 'fighters' all came from poor and enormous families with thirty plus siblings. They feel that what spoiled their future was their parents' and particularly their fathers' total disregard for their lives or futures. These young Ivorian or Liberian young men are easily seduced to join a rebel force that has guns like they see on TV or movies about American Gangsters. Sha, a young Ivorian told Packer that after the war, he wanted to go to New York, become a Marine, learn to fly helicopters and use heavy weapons. Then while drinking heavily another young man Romeo says to Packer, "If you can't pay the young stuff (him), the war will enter America---let me tell you today. Because you don't give them money. The man we want to see is **bin Laden.** We want to see him, to join him. Because he can pay revolutionaries." (p76).

Fatherless hungry young men. Packer saw had tee shirts with Bush and bin Laden's pictures side by side. In the face of being abandoned by mothers and fathers these young people find heroes in American pop celebrities, local warlords, gangsters or political demagogues. Yul, a young Ivorian man said to Packer after a struggle to get an 'Identity Card, requiring a 'Certificate of Loss': "A man must have a father at his side to help him. If he doesn't—Who's going to help me? Who? I don't see." (p77).

Packer spots this as an effort to find an identity in a place that has no use for them. These young people's search for prowess, strength and possibly **Negative Identity (Erikson, 1964 p97-99*****).** African young adults' parent-hunger and search for identity in 'all the wrong places and faces' should be of major concern to any American. If my patient Tommy's mother was failing him regarding guidance about media violence, how much more concern should we have for these struggling young people in Africa. **911** underline for us all, the fact that these young Ivoirians are not that far away from America. Yule and Tommy are not totally different psychologically. Tommy and his mother were fortunate to find therapy help.

'Smart bombs' and bullets will not win the 'War on terror'. Victory over terror and violence can only occur in battles for the Mind and Heart. Can we mobilize a rejuvenated and modernized Peace Corps" forty years after President Kennedy gave it birth?

*** Negative Identity is a 'debased self-image and role', resulting from lack of social contact and continuity via adult healthy, caring role models.

References:

*   McLuhan, M. UNDERSTADING MEDIA: THE EXTENSIONS OF MAN. (1964) New York McGraw-Hill Company.

**   Olsson, P. "The Terrorist and the Terrorized" in THE PSYCHODYNAMIC OF INTERNATIONAL RELATIONSHIPS Vol. I Chap.14, Ed by Volkan, Julius & Montville. Lexington Books. D.C. Heath and Company? Lexington, Massachusetts/Toronto, p181

* * * American Academy of Child & Adolescent Psychiatry, Facts for Families # 13, 2003.

**** Packer, G. "Gangsta War: Young fighters take their lead from American pop culture", THE NEW YORKER November3, 2003.

****Erikson, E. (1964) INSIGHT AND RESPONSIBILITY, New York, W.W. Norton & Company.

LESSONS LEARNED FROM THERAPY WORK WITH TOMMY AND HIS MOM

Dr. Tolman's Notes:

I learned from Tommy's treatment that if one or both parents have significant mental or personality problems treatment of both parent and child is optimal, often essential. It is a rare exception for a child to receive successful treatment without their parent's cooperation. Often when a child is sent or brought to therapy they really are a designated patient representing a cry for help by the whole family system. Another stark lesson I learned from Tommy and his mom is that not only children are affected negatively by TV violence. Adults personalities can be warped and damaged by TV violence and Hollywood-portrayed irresponsible sexual behaviors. Finally, unusual occurrences and psychological afflictions found in psychotherapy patients reflect and provide entree into exploring societal dilemmas and their resolution. Many important therapy cases trigger important clinical contributions to the psychiatric literature.

5—A BOY WHO WANTED TO BE IN PRISON

Billy Furst pressed his nose against the window. He loved to dream about climbing out the window and running off to be a cowboy on a ranch far away from the city. Billy however shared a room with two other boys. At least he had the single bed and not the bunk bed. This foster home was called the Bunkhouse. Billy guessed this place was called Bunkhouse, because the house dad and owner, Mr. Clark, always wore a black cowboy hat and black cowboy boots. Sometimes to keep from crying Billy thinks to himself a lot.

The Bunkhouse mom gave me a small chocolate cake today. It had twelve candles on it. Bunkhouse mom is nice. I ate it after breakfast so the Bunkhouse mates wouldn't eat it all. The cake tasted so good! My Bunkhouse mate Joey scares me. He would have grabbed my cake and eaten it. Then Joey would laugh his mean laugh. If I cussed him he would punch me hard. In a spot, the Bunkhouse mother wouldn't notice. If I ever cried, Joey would get even meaner. Like with that Howe kid who went to another place after Joey broke his arm. Henry didn't tattle, but everyone knew what happened. I would only want to go away from the Bunkhouse if I could be with my dad.

****

Juanita Clark sat waiting for Billy's appointment with Dr. Tom Tolman. Juanita and her husband John couldn't have kids of their own. Juanita figured her eggs had been too old and not good enough to make a baby. It was John's idea that they should start a foster home. John said they could call it The Bunkhouse. John smiled big at that idea. They could get money from the state for every boy they kept at their place.

Juanita also knew that John knew how much she wanted kids. She loved John for his knowing that without her saying it. Juanita knew that deep down John wanted a place for kids that would be like Cal Farley's ranch where John grew up. John once said that he probably would have ended up in Huntsville state prison if it hadn't been for old' Cal Farley. John was tough but fair with their boys.

Juanita and John didn't take their boys to a psychiatrist often but John had caught Billy stealing cash from his wallet. Juanita found one of her missing gold rings in Billy's locker when they had to do a room search. They didn't like doing room searches because the boys deserved privacy, but sometimes it had to be done. Billy's school teacher caught him stealing candy from her desk and called Juanita. The teacher said she like Billy and wished he could get help. Billy got caught stealing food from the grocery store. The owner who caught him said he would have given food to Billy but had to tell her when Billy stole it.

Billy looked sad and said he was sorry. He only wanted food and money for his trip. Juanita sensed Billy was telling it straight but he wouldn't say where he intended to go on his trip. They, of course, had many of their boys run away, but usually not as young as Billy. She and John hadn't felt angry at Billy. They really wanted to get him help.

****

Tom Tolman MD enjoyed working with kids who were verbal enough and smart enough to use therapy to help themselves. Billy Furst was his first evaluation for the day. Tom read the referring school psychologist's referral note and preliminary diagnosis. The note was concise:

> Ten-year-old slender boy. He has stolen money and valuable objects at his
> foster home and at school. Billy even stole food at the neighborhood grocery

saying he needed it for a trip. Billy didn't specify the destination of his trip. Preliminary diagnosis, Kleptomania. Possible antisocial personality with criminal behavior.

Billy's housemother described Billy's troubled behavior in detail. Tolman immediately liked Juanita Clark. She looked Tom directly in the eye and clearly liked Billy in a sincere way. Tom could tell this from her voice tone and eyes. Sincerity was not easy to detect and never quantifiable, but Juanita Clark had it. She described The Bunkhouse and the other kids living there. She described Billy as quiet and shy but friendly with the other boys in the house except a fellow named Joey. No one got along with well with Joey.

"Joey is our angry problem boy. He's hard to like but so are many of the boys we get from cruel and abusive family situations. My husband John is the only one Joey seems to trust because John spends time with him like he does with all the boys. Joey always wants more and more attention but John is firm about stuff like that. Joey respects him as do all our boys."

Mrs. Clark didn't know much about Billy's childhood except that the court social worker told her that placement was necessary because Billy's father shot and killed Billy's mother. Billy was an only child and had been at the Bunkhouse for about five months. She wished Billy could stay with them but the stealing had to stop. She did say that Billy liked to read and drew some interesting and well-done pictures. Tolman thanked Mrs. Clark for the information and said that he would like to meet with her and her husband sometimes as a part of Billy's treatment. The rest of the hour he would spend starting to get to know Billy.

Billy had deep blue eyes and a sad but alert expression. Tolman thought about how to begin their talk. But Billy abruptly started their conversation by commenting, "Gee, what a lot of books you have."

Tom invited Billy to look at them. Billy walked over to the shelves and looked at titles. He picked out one titled, *Parenthood.* Billy said, "I don't have parents around anymore."

Billy then grabbed a book about "The Cowboy and American Culture." Billy said, "I like cowboys and rodeos. My dad was a cowboy bull rider in rodeos before he got hurt and had to work at his gas station. He took me to a rodeo once at the Astrodome. Once when I was with him at his gas station he said he missed rodeoing. He said the gas station took up all his time. Now, he's in prison all the time. They say he got put there because he killed my mother. I don't believe he did. I wish mom and dad were still with me."

Tolman asked Billy, "What do you remember about your mom and dad?"

Billy said, "When I was little we were happy. We had picnics in Hermann Park or Memorial Park. Then Daddy got hurt and had to work all the time at his gas station. Mom got crying a lot, she said because Daddy wasn't around. They both drank too much beer when Daddy was around. He mainly watched football and rodeo on TV. They yelled a lot. That scared me."

Tolman told Billy they would talk more about his parents and other things on his mind at their next therapy talk. The time was over for today.

Tolman valued the 5-10 minutes before and after therapy sessions. His random thoughts focused between the lines and spoken words. Tom had learned to pay careful attention to his feelings during that precious time. It was a part of the session as much as the words with his patient.

I like Billy. I like and trust Juanita Clark. I feel she and John Clark are good and sincere souls. I'm fascinated by the assessment of a person's sincerity. It seems to cluster around a trio of trust. Truth and trust go together when it comes to assessing sincerity. Truth and trust over time are the bedrocks of successful psychotherapy. Billy's sincerity stems from a Billy Budd type innocence that hadn't quite been crushed by disappointments in adults—yet. Tolman noted that Billy couldn't in his account be convinced that his dad killed his mother.

Billy, like many depressed and abandoned kids talked like a little adult. Such pseudo adulthood had two sides. One was the ability of Tolman to do talking therapy with Billy; the other was that progress in therapy would mean Billy could just be a twelve-year-old kid again and not a sad little adult before his time.

I didn't even talk to Billy about his stealing. Why? Sometimes things that are not talked about in therapy are the most important What is Billy's kleptomania about? Money, food and a gold ring belonging to his house mother. Her ring to sell? Or, to remember her with while on his trip? Billy had mentioned a trip to somewhere. Where? Why?

Juanita's sincerity stemmed from her direct eye contact and as the old expression goes, her actions toward Billy spoke volumes more than her words.

Tolman made some quick notes and went out to greet his next patient. The fact that he hadn't talked to Billy about his stealing perplexed Tolman, but it must be important.

****

In his dream Billy was little, much younger. The same scary things happened over-and-over like a scary TV movie that he was forced to watch. In the dream, Mom was getting more and drunk. She was crying quietly. The phone rang and Billy, like always in the dream, heard his mom say, "Jason, I got to see you... Yeah, The Blue Moon. It's right down the street so Billy will be okay here while I'm gone for a while." [Note: Name change to Jason—you may have a better one, but a Jake was in a previous story.]

After his mom leaves Daddy came home. He had beer breath and says, "Where is your mother?"

Billy hesitates. Daddy grabs him demanding to know. Daddy's face is real mean looking. Billy blurts out, "She said, Blue Moon."

Hank Furst rushes out. Billy hears Daddy's truck door slam. Like always in the dream Billy looks out the trailer window and sees his daddy heading down the street toward the Blue Moon with his big .45 revolver tucked in his belt near his back pocket. Then the three loud shots—BAM, BAM, and BAM! Then he hears the sirens again.

Billy wakes up was sweating and scared. The rain on the window gradually helped him get back to a light sleep.

****

I like Dr. Tolman. Going to him is hard but, he listens as hard and good as the Bunkhouse mom and dad. I hope he can help me stop feeling so sad. I guess I got to try hard not to steal stuff for a little while to see if Dr. T can help me. Anyway, I got to get a map to figure out how to get to

Huntsville anyway. I'm scared Dr. T thinks my dad is a murderer and bad guy. I hope he doesn't hate my dad. Daddy must have had to shoot to protect himself. Mom would get real mad when she got drunk. Her man friend, Jason, smiled a lot, but he talked mean when he drank beer too. So, did Daddy sometimes get mean?

Billy seemed eager to see Tom Tolman. But this time Billy was quiet, yet, looking eager. He was glancing over at Tom's book shelves.

"Billy, what do you like to read?"

"Cowboys, all about cowboys."

"Last time at our talk you said your father was a cowboy and he took you to a rodeo. Tell me more about your daddy."

As Billy's eyes, teared-up he said, "Daddy was a bull riding cowboy till he got hurt. Then he bought a gas station. I miss my Daddy and my Mom. I have a scary dream about Mom and Daddy. I had it last night. It's the same every time."

Billy told Tom the dream as tears ran down his cheeks. "Daddy is all I have left. I'm saving enough money and food to go see him. I don't care if I get put in jail for stealing because I might be sent to the same prison as Daddy.

Now Tolman knew what the stealing was about. What to do? What to say? Tom went with his gut.

"Billy, I think you and I need to write letters to your dad. Let him know you miss him and want to see him. Do you want to do that? If you say "yes," I want your permission to call your dad and let him know our letters will be coming."

Billy stopped his tears as he nodded affirmatively. They spent the rest of the session and part of the next session writing down things to say. Between sessions Billy drew a good picture of a cowboy and the bunkhouse where he lived.

Tolman sent a letter to Hank Furst, care of Huntsville State Prison. Hank had not answered so Tom called the warden's office, explained who he was and asked how to call Hank Furst. The clerk looked up Furst's exercise period and suggested Tom might call during that time frame. Tom wanted to contact Hank before Tom's next session with Billy.

The cellblock phone where Hank Furst was incarcerated at Huntsville State Prison rang a dozen times before rough voice answered.

"Sullivan here, who are you?"

Tom asked for Hank Furst. Hank came to the phone and Tolman explained who he was and why he wanted to send him Billy's letters. Hank said gruffly,

"Why in hell do you want to do that Doc?"

"Because Billy misses you and says he wants to write to you. Billy has been stealing stuff and probably does worse things because he thinks he could get to see you and be with you in prison. He's staying at a foster home and you're all the family he knows."

There was a long silence before Hank said, "Hell Doc, do you know that I shot his mother and her damn boyfriend?"

"I know that and Billy believes you had to have good reason to shoot to protect yourself."

Furst went on, "That bastard boyfriend of hers had a knife and she was swinging a beer bottle. Look Doc, I can write but I wouldn't know what to say. Hell, go ahead and send them. I've been talking to a priest here and maybe he could help me with it."

"I'm glad you're talking to the priest. Billy and I will be sending the letter this week."

Tom got the accurate mailing address, the priest's name and agreed to follow-up with Hank by phone and letter soon.

Billy agreed and was excited as they walked to a mailbox near the clinic and Billy put the letter through the slot. So, began a steady correspondence between Billy and his dad. Slowly as Billy learned the accumulating doses of truth from his dad his urges to join his dad in prison ceased but Billy talked about visiting as soon as it was possible. Tom was touched by a father's efforts at loving epistles from prison. Billy shed many more tears as he and Tolman read the letters and explored Billy's feelings, fears and anger. Father Lawson told Tom that many tears and pounded fists on a stuffed chair occurred as he and Hank read the letters and wrote return letters. Hank put pictures of Billy and Billy's pictures on the walls of his cell. In his letters, Hank Furst wrote poignantly about the importance of anger control that he had learned too late. He beseeched Billy to learn that and stick with school which Hank had himself neglected.

Billy began to work steadily in his psychotherapy with Tolman. After resolving his separation anxiety and father hunger, Billy had grieved the loss of his mother. Through his letters, Hank Furst had shared his prayerful search for forgiveness about the killing of his wife and her boyfriend Jake. The prison priest father Lawson had written to Billy about Billy's father's prayers asking for God's forgiveness. Billy read library books about Catholicism, prayer and forgiveness. Billy chose to attend an Episcopalian church with friends where they enjoyed activities and discussions with a youth minister and his wife.

Billy began to make other friends at school and help other newly arriving kids at the Bunkhouse. Billy met his first girlfriend and struggled with ordinary adolescent issues about intimacy, rejection, acne and plans about saving for college. Billy found an after-school job.

Billy had gone with John and Juanita Clark to visit his dad Hank at Huntsville for the first time. The Clarks and Billy met with father Lawson and Hank Furst. Father Lawson confirmed Hank's positive activities at the prison library where he worked and studied at a college level after finishing a high school equivalency exam. Hanks letters to Billy continued. According to the Clark's it had gone well.

Tom Tolman's journal notes:

Sometimes it is a joy to find and work with foster parents like Juanita and John Clark. It is moving to see rare examples of resilience and triumphs of the human spirit like I discovered working with Billy, his dad, father Lawson, and the Clarks. There are so many other situations where bitterness, unresolved grief, resentment and hate to lead a kid down a trail to crime and prison.

[Note: suggest that the following text be incorporated in to Tom's journal notes and the heading below deleted. Or, alternately, the journal notes be incorporated into the "Lessons Learned section]

LESSONS LEARNED FROM BILLY FURST'S PSYCHOTHERAPY.

Tom Tolman's notes: Some foster parents are good and special souls. They are often unsung heroes because the stability and help they provide for youths goes without formal recognition. Attachment problems among abused, orphaned, adopted or abandoned kids is a serious and common problem. It helps immensely if the kids have surrogate parents who care and are effective at parenting. Billy's father impressed me with the fact that some criminals that commit serious crimes like murder can find forms of healing and redemption.

6—A BOY WHO WAS A WOULD-BE BOMBER

Houston in early August is like a cross between a pizza oven and a steam cleaner. Ben Hughes was stunned at the contrast between Middlebury Vermont and Rice University's home city. As a junior transfer student from Middlebury, Ben had looked forward to the rigorous engineering courses he planned to pack into his final two undergraduate years. The challenge now he though was Houston's infernal heat and a Redneck roommate named Tug Smith. He pulled out the journal that he kept hidden in the back of his desk drawer and began to write.

August 15 – I'm damn mad and scared. I heard of rednecks in places like Texas, but not at Rice University, the Harvard of the South. Of all the screwed-up things to encounter here, I get Tug Smith for a roommate. In addition to being a redneck, Smith also seems to be a queer. He smiles at me and tried to hug me when I got advanced placement in upper division math courses. He says he comes from a family of huggers. That's BS. Since he thinks I live so far from home, Tug wants me to go home with him to Jasper Texas for Thanksgiving. Never! If the sucker touches me one more time I'll hit him hard and hurt him. I learned long ago that you got to be the first one to punch when you're seriously threatened and in danger.

Tried to discuss the situation with our dorm advisor, Dr. Maxwell, but all he said was that all roommates take a while to adjust to each other. He probably says that to all new students. I'm NOT going to adjust to Tug Smith, PERIOD! Tug, what a fag name anyway. And here at Rice they call the dorms "houses" and the advisors are called "Masters." Guess that's why Maxwell gives such crappy advice.

August 28 – I can't sleep because my damn roomie stays up late listening to country music while he studies. I study in the library, but when I come home late he says he turns the music down, but not really. I've been dreaming about smashing guitars and banjos. Tug says good night to me in some soft, gay fag way. Damn, why didn't I get a football player for a roommate. At Middlebury, I had a room by myself.

September 17 – *Okay, I have tried for a month now. I confronted Tug nicely about his damn music and his smarmy style but he laughed. I didn't hit him but he's really pissing me off more and more.*

September 30 – *I made a pipe bomb to put under his car. If I must, I'll use it. As a chemistry and physics major, I know about bombs. A pipe bomb can be set up to blow and hurt him bad as soon as he starts his car. It won't kill him—just teach him a lesson. I'm going to talk to Dr. Maxwell once more before I blow it up. I won't be dominated by a fag!*

****

[Note: Tom is now back in his first year as a psychiatry resident—in previous stories he is in practice and a supervising doctor. Do you see this story as fitting in earlier in chronological order? It makes some sense to have Tom grow over the years introducing him as a young doctor and then a more experienced practitioner. On the other hand, you might prefer the stories in the current order for impact – something to think about.]

Dr. Tom Tolman was doing well as a first-year psychiatry resident at Baylor Med School. During the second half of the year he was supposed to find and evaluate a bright, verbally competent patient who he would then see in psychodynamic psychotherapy two to three times a week for the duration of his three-year residency. Tolman would have weekly psychotherapy supervision by a senior staff psychiatrist. He had found children to see twice weekly but still needed several adult or young adult therapy cases to facilitate his learning to do intensive psychotherapy. Tom was excited about this new domain of psychiatry work. His first patient at the Baylor outpatient clinic was a Rice University student referred for evaluation by his dorm advisor Dr. Carl Maxwell. Maxwell said in the referral note, "Highly anxious transfer student with severe problems adjusting to his roommate."

Good, a bright Rice student to work with in long-term psychotherapy. According to the textbooks, psychodynamic psychotherapy is the treatment of choice for a bright, verbal patient with anxiety disorder.

****

Ben Hughes sat in the waiting room chair, his legs bouncing constantly. When Tolman called his name, Ben looked around furtively to see if he noticed anyone who knew him from school. After all, Rice University was right across Fannin and Main Streets from the Baylor Medical School clinic. Ben abruptly leaped up and followed close behind Tolman as they entered Tolman's clinic office. Ben was perspiring, mildly shaky and trembling. Tolman thought he looked intense and eager to talk to someone.

Tolman asked Ben why he had come to the clinic. Ben stuttered a bit as he said, "I'm afraid I will hurt my roommate, maybe have to kill him."

My God, and I thought this case was going to be a good long-term psychotherapy case. But, someone could be in immediate danger here! Do I hospitalize Ben immediately?

Ben stammered as he talked quickly. Tolman listened carefully to Ben describe his roommate Tug Smith—Tug's "hugging habits," his smarmy lilting voice, and his fear that Tug was a homosexual with amorous designs.

I like Ben. But I'm scared. Yet I feel strangely comfortable listening to Ben. He has an innocent Billy Budd, Vermont country boy quality. He seems ready to talk, not act. The books talk about a "therapeutic contract. How can I establish a contract and safe domain for us to work together in therapy?

Tolman tried to screw up his confidence level saying, "Ben, I want to work with you in psychotherapy but have to feel that things are safe for us to work together. I need to see you for an hour, three times a week, and with your permission, I need to contact Dr. Maxwell.to see if a single room is available for you or at least a change of roommates. I will ask Dr. Maxwell to talk to Tug Smith about not pushing a friendship with you now. You also must disassemble the pipe bomb and safely dispose of it immediately. I also want to prescribe a calming medication so you can sleep and keep up with your studies. What are your thoughts about that plan?"

Ben thought for a minute. Tolman noticed that Ben became less tremulous and his legs bounced up and down less frequently. "Yea, I like that plan and hope I can switch rooms very soon. How long do I need to see you? How much will this treatment cost? I don't want my dad to know about this and I know he wouldn't pay for it."

Tom told Ben that they needed to work at his therapy long enough for him to feel more comfortable and confident in his relationships and at school. The clinic had a sliding scale and his Rice student insurance and his co-pay would cover the costs. Together they would decide on the goals, review how the treatment was going and how long it would last. Ben seemed satisfied. They set up meeting times for each Monday, Wednesday and Friday. Tom gave Ben a prescription and discussed side effects and benefits he hoped Ben would get from the tranquilizer.

Ben seemed slightly less anxious and tense when he arrived for his session the next Friday. I got rid of the bomb 'for now.' I'm sleeping better. Dr. Tolman, thank you, I really needed the rest and Maxwell found a single room for me. It's cramped but comfortable enough to study there. I've only seen Tug once since I left and he was too friendly, but less intense. I glared at him hoping he would notice."

Tolman was relieved. Ben also was less intense. Tom knew that soon he would need to discuss Ben's experiences with his friends.

Ben continued, "So far, I notice the kids in my classes are serious about the subjects and I don't spot any fags. I never was afraid of fags in high school or Middlebury College. I sort of miss Middlebury. It was close to my parent's farm and a couple of my friends would come to our farm and dad would pay us to pitch hay and do work. Dad did make fun of one friend who was slow in his work. Dad asked me if he was a fag or just a sissy. I told dad he was music major and didn't want to risk blisters on his piano playing hands."

Tom asked Ben about his dad and their farm. "Grandpa Hughes, my father's father bought and worked the Hughes farm near Rutland Vermont all his life. My dad inherited the farm and still works it. We have cows, chickens, pigs, and grow corn and cabbage. My father's name is Hank. He's tall, strong and doesn't say much. My mother Sophie says, 'Hank Hughes, you only know dawn till dusk work.' Mom makes dad go out to dinner and a movie once a month. Dad gripes about it but seems to secretly enjoy it."

"Tell me about your relationship with your dad."

Ben gave a cryptic reply, "Dad seems to like it when we work hard together on the farm. We talk only about the work we're doing. I think dad is disappointed, probably mad, that I decided to study aeronautical engineering and not farming. Dad said, 'what you gonna be, a crop duster?' He hasn't talked about my studies since. He doesn't say it, but I think he is disappointed that he didn't have any other kids, especially another son who could work the farm and keep the Hughes farm going."

Ben spent the rest of the session talking in detail about his math, physics and chemistry professors. He was only concerned about his organic chemistry professor who he described as having a [fogy] [Note: fogy – m. old fashioned or "faggy" – not a real word according to the dictionary but in quotes could be used if that's what Ben wants?] voice. Ben talked right up till the end of the hour and seemed eager to meet the next Monday.

Tom spent some time taking a few notes and having free-floating thoughts about their first psychotherapy session. *Ben seemed much less tense and I feel really relieved about his getting that bomb out of the picture. I trust him about that even though he qualified it with the words, 'for now.'*

Tolman's psychotherapy supervisor Shane West seemed slightly wary when Tom told him about his first session with Ben.

"Tom, I like the way you searched your own intuitions and inner hunches about Hughes. It's good you've scheduled three sessions per week with Ben. With three sessions, a week we can keep an eye out for trouble like missed sessions, further violent fantasy, or dreams of situations with violent resolutions."

During the next three months Ben described the social isolation he experiences in both his childhood and now in his adolescence. Tolman and West agreed that the description that Ben provided about his two close friendships revealed his empathy toward his friends' difficulties.

Ben described very inhibited efforts at individual dating and several "group dates" to dances and football games.

Ben began to bring up Tug Smith again. Tug had not sought contact with Ben, rather, Ben began to dream about fight scenes and wrestling matches between him and Tug where he held Tug down and pinned him.

Then Ben came to a session sweating, pale, and noticeably trembling. "Dr. Tolman I promised you no bombs, but last night I dreamed I made one to blow-up Tug. I'm scared. Tug had a weird smile and I could smell his Old Spice cologne. Yuck!"

Tolman asked calmly, "Tell me more about your dream and what went on yesterday. Events that happened the day before might connect with something in your dream. Take a deep breath, relax, and let your mind wander through your day yesterday. Close your eyes if it helps."

Ben's shoulders slumped as he closed his eyes and leaned back in his chair. "I aced a chemistry test. I worked with weights at the gym. I walked by the football practice field. The coach was working the guys hard in the hot sun. They were sweating. I thought they must be looking forward to a nice shower. I started to study at my new room and my father called. He hurt his back while pitching hay. He said he sure wished I was there to do work. I got tense and told him I had to study." Ben sat silently for several minutes.

Tolman broke the silence. "Athletes sweating, wrestling in your dream, what about the Old Spice smell in the dream?"

Ben stiffened, sat up straight, stared straight at Tolman and said, "My dad uses Old Spice after shave. The last time I smelled that was after my bomb blew up in our barn my senior year in high school."

Ben looked down and began to cry quietly, "I hated that Mr. Evans my physics teacher. He was mean to lots of us but he had a hard-on for me. He made fun of me once when I didn't get an A on a test. He kept me after school to give me special advanced tutoring. Hell, I could have tutored that bald fag. He would get that fag voice and put his arm on my shoulder sometimes. He said he would get me ready for MIT. It made me feel creepy when he did that. I told father and he just laughed and kept working. Father said, 'You can handle that Ben boy.'"

Ben wiped his nose with Kleenex and continued, "Doc Tolman, that's when I began to study bomb-making. It was easy and each night when I worked on it in the barn I felt stronger about not being suckered and hugged by Evans. The hate I was filled with gave me more power and feeling in control. Then one night as I was mixing up some concentrated gunpowder in my large mortar with a pestle...the whole thing blew—BAM!"

Ben slammed the desk with his hand. He showed Tolman some scars and a slightly deformed finger on his right hand. "I've got scars in my crotch right next to my pecker and nuts. My father heard the blast and came out to the barn. He saw me stunned and bleeding. Dad picked me up in his arms and carried me to the truck as he yelled to mom to start it up. Dad held me and put pressure on the wounds all the way to the hospital. I can still smell dad's Old Spice after shave and feel his strong arms around me. Dr. Tolman, that's the only time I can remember my dad holding me."

Ben used more tissue and they sat in silence for several minutes. "Ben, Tug Smith triggered important but painful memories and unresolved conflicts in your mind. As we work to resolve these issues within you, your inner strengths will grow. Your confidence in yourself will make bomb-making unnecessary."

Ben breathed deeply and stretched in his chair. He talked about his increasing awareness of his anger at his father saying, "Father doesn't help me with any money for school, other than money I make working at the farm."

Ben tensed up and pounded his deformed hand on the arm of his chair. Tolman knew to let Ben continue to ventilate as Ben talked about his father and their "Vince Lombardi relationship" as Ben called it. Ben talked more about the problems he had socially during high school. His father wouldn't let him use the farm truck to go on dates or to parties. Ben double-dated with friends who kidded him, but tried to be helpful. Tolman said something about people wanting to help him—even Tug Smith. Ben disagreed but spent the rest of the session talking about his father. "You know, Doc, I never told my father what exploded in the barn—and he never asked me or brought up the subject."

****

Tom and his supervisor Shane West agreed that Tom's previous session with Ben had been a crucial one and was pivotal for success in Ben's treatment. And, it was. Tom saw Ben for psychotherapy sessions two to three times per week for the next two and a half years. Their closeness developed steadily, and the trusting depth of their work together allowed Ben to explore his insecurity about his masculinity. He gradually saw that his bomb making was a cry for help rather than a powerful protective tool. Their sessions were tense as Tolman confronted

Ben's angry paranoia about fags and queers. Such defensiveness was really about Ben's fear of closeness with men was really about closeness with people in general. Work on the connection of this issue to Ben's sexual identity was crucial and continued over many months of work.

At one point in the therapy process, Ben had a dream about Tolman being bisexual or homosexual. Ben was terrified—but fearfully shared the dream with Tolman. Work with that dream helped Ben to see connections to his father's stilted relationships with women and that his father's macho controlling, dominating style was really a poor role-model. Ben began to understand that machoism and fag-bashing were not really masculine but defensive. Ben felt close to his mother who clearly loved both Ben and his father, but Ben acknowledged that she was too demur and should have stood up more to his father.

In his dating efforts Ben was very anxious and at first, choosing passive but good students who were classmates. Such women admired his intellect but in time Ben also valued "girls with spunk" who couldn't be readily dominated. Ben's social confidence and competence grew steadily because of his many, many months of psychotherapy work.

Ben eventually was no longer felt threatened and became comfortable with occasionally studying with several homosexual classmates. He could still be friends and colleagues with people who were homosexual. After the initial sparks, several crucial confrontations during summer breaks brought Ben and his father. During his final year at Rice Ben received several honors and prestigious grad-school scholarships. His father attended the graduation and shook hands vigorously with Ben.

Tom Tolman attended the graduation and Ben took obvious pleasure in introducing Tom to his dad, his girlfriend, and his friend, Tug Smith.

In a Christmas note to Tolman, Ben quipped, "Having a blast here at MIT, but, the good kind."

LESSONS LEARNED FROM BEN HUGHES' PSYCHOTHERAPY

Tom Tolman's notes: Assessment of potential violence and suicide is a humbling and challenging arena in clinical psychotherapy work. Ben helped me to pay attention to the quiet inner voice of intuition and accurate empathy. Monday mornings provide many smug quarterbacks. But not so, in the process of psychotherapy 's here-and-now world. No twenty-twenty hindsight found. Such an uncertain work-world does provide excitement, fear, challenges and intense rewards.

7—A BOY ABANDONED: LUIS'S SANCTUARY

[Note: You sure got me here! I was seeing "Victor" so clearly being real. Wonderful depiction.]

Luis wanted to be warm, happy, and able to smile—like the people driving by the corner of Cesar Chavez and Congress Avenue, and nearby streets. It was a partly sunny in Austin today, but December and now January had been cold. At night, Luis' two old wool blankets didn't keep him warm enough. At least the bugs were not bad so the grass and leaves near the freeway bridge helped with warmth.

"Wipe that crooked smile off your face kid! Get off my money spot Mex. "

Damn, it was big Red! As the down-in-their-luckers called him. When Red said to get off his begging turf, you did it. If you didn't, Red would find you at the night camp areas and beat you bloody. One night, Red kicked Luis as he slept. Luis had limped for weeks till the bruise went away.

Luis thinks cold sweaty thoughts about something else—*Red is scary, but nothing compared to Victor. Thank God Victor hasn't come after me lately.*

Luis quickly moved away towards another street corner. The Austin cops basically looked the other way unless the "down-in-their luckers," got into fights. If the luckers got too close to their cars, the smiley people frowned. They got scared, and called in complaints to the police on their car phones. The street rules for luckers in Austin were simple, clear and rigid. Fights out on the street corners were taboo because fights and overly aggressive begging meant no money from the smiley people in their shiny new cars. Victor's voice once boomed saying, "The smiley people in the shiny cars got to be treated really careful. Their damn guilt is a fragile thing. They got jobs and money but somehow know deep down, that a string of bad breaks could land them on our street or worse."

Victor said that someday soon, even in rich Texas, more and more people would join the ranks of the down-in-their luckers. Especially hit would be those without a high school education or the new herds of pot smokers and other druggies. Victor said the government doesn't want to pay to feed potheads for years in their prisons anymore.

So, Victor cautioned further, saying, "When they give you money they are paying the big guilt-man, with a capital G. Don't scare me, but don't look, act, or be so happy either. Damn, Luis, I call it 'artful pitifulness.'" Then, Victor laughed his angry mocking laugh. Luis felt cold chills.

Luis hoped that by the end of the day he would have enough money to afford a motel room where he could take a bath this week. Then he could stop by St. Mary's and put a donation in the offering box. Maybe even see Sister Laura. Her smile was like a tiny glimpse of heaven. But, Luis just couldn't let Victor see him make an offering or there would be literal hell to pay.

Luis and scary Victor had gone to St. Mary's school together years ago. Vic enjoyed beating up other boys after school. Sister Laura stopped the fights when she could. Vic had hated Sister Laura because he said she smiled too much. And, not at him.

Yesterday Luis collected twelve dollars from the happy smiling car people. Today no luck by late afternoon. Luis didn't receive any money and few car people smiled or even looked at him. The cold breeze bit into his face and through his tattered cloth jacket. Red had stolen Luis's thicker warm fleece last spring. Red claimed that he had seen the jacket first in the ditch.

The wet things started streaming down his cold cheeks and Luis started to cough and spit up those green and yellow gobs.

Luis feared what lay ahead. He was afraid the typical sequence was about to occur. First, the severe nervousness, then the body tension, and then the terrible confused crooked thinking. The crooked thoughts prevented him from finding the places he needed to go for protection. Then finally, came the need-fear dilemma of Victor's presence—that earthquake voice. The voice Luis could feel, taste, smell, see, and touch. The power voice looked like a tornado made of whirling blood, spit and dust. It was the size of a pick- up truck that could run over him at dizzying speed. The voice smelled like puke and sweat with a taste like cooked garlic, hot sauce and onions

Luis's parents died in a car crash when he was twelve. Sister Laura knew Luis because she worked at the Catholic children's home and school. Luis, an only child with no known relatives, had been sent to St. Mary's after his parents died. Sister Laura treated all the kids at St. Mary's Home like they were her own children. She seemed especially kind and gentle to Luis.

Recently, Luis refused Sister's offer of the free shelter. Ever since Luis lost the church janitor job at St. Mary's several years ago, he felt too ashamed to accept charity. Especially from Sister Laura, who he had always loved.

Lucker camps in Austin are located under bridges, near isolated dry streambeds, and in dense underbrush at the sides of freeways near bridges. The shelter of the nearby bridges is essential in the event of rain or snow. Some luckers have plastic covers they use because trying to claim shelter under a bridge after a rain has started can lead to a beating from the lord of that turf. Luis and other luckers know they can't go to the camps to sleep until after it gets dark. This poses problems because in the near dark it gets hard to spot territories staked out by bullies like big Red. Settling in too close to Red's claim could result in a beating. If a guy or gal lucker had a bottle of booze or sometimes their body to share with Red, he might allow them to stay for the night in relative peace. It worked best if Red got real drunk and the lucker left Red's camp before day light.

Just before Luis got to the bridge area where he might find a place to put his bedroll and stuff down. Victor's voice boomed so loud that Luis's head vibrated. "You sniveling bastard, no sleep for you tonight! I got a place for you but you got to walk a long way. See that parking lot of the HEB? Get one of those grocery carts to put your stuff in and listen to my directions sucker."

Luis did as he was told. Victor commanded him to keep walking along the service road beside US 35 south. He used an old towel to keep his hands warm as he walked all night. Luis's few possessions were not heavy except the sturdy fry pan he got years ago at a St. Mary's tag sale. It had come in handy one night when he drove off an angry drunken Red. Luis used to cook eggs or fish in it sometimes. Just before sun up, Luis nearing exhaustion and in a rare act of defiance, yelled, "Damn, Victor, where do you want me to go?"

Victor replied, "Don't cuss me sucker lucker! Ha, Ha, Ha, Ha!! A mile further, you will see a big strong building marked with a big sign with big red circles that look like that archery target at church camp. Even you can't miss it. Go in there, wash up and I'll talk at you later. Don't get in trouble punk."

Luis did as he was told. He left his grocery cart full of his things behind a dumpster outside the big red circle fortress. He only took his towel and toothbrush. The place had its own big red grocery carts. Luis took one to walk around with and placed his towel, soap and

toothbrush in it. At six a.m., there were only a few people in the place and none of them were

smilers or luckers. One guy with a bright red shirt scowled and looked at Luis with suspicion.

Luis wasn't scared because Victor had commanded him to be here.

Luis was amazed at this red circle friendly fortress. After he washed up in the restroom,

he noticed that this place had all kinds of wonderful things for guests. There was milk, cereal,

fruit and vegetables. Luis found a cereal bowl, a spoon and even some napkins. He took them to

a chair in one of the isles. He enjoyed a good breakfast and then washed his bowl and spoon. He

started exploring the rest of this special new place. He got a new toothbrush and toothpaste. Luis

spotted a smooth warm new fleece jacket and put it in his cart. He smiled and said to himself,

"Eat your heart out Red!"

Then Luis put a long sharp carving knife in his cart. He might need it with guys like Red.

The pistols and rifles were probably locked up somewhere. A twenty-two or bow and arrow

would allow him to hunt squirrels or rabbits but he couldn't locate them. He placed a small

tackle box, some fishing lures, hooks, bobbers and a fishing knife in his cart.

Luis moved leisurely toward the men's clothes section. A loud crying baby and her loud

talking mother came towards him. Luis made a shushing gesture across his mouth with his index

finger. Rather than being relieved and quiet, the women quickly hurried away toward the front

door. Victor wasn't talking yet as Luis walked past an older couple looking at bath towels. They

smiled at him until Luis gestured for them to be silent. Then they looked puzzled. If too much

talking and too much smiling happened right now, Victor's voice would come blasting back in his ears and at everyone in this new place. Luis didn't want everyone in this nice place to be scared and confused like he was getting. He hated his jumbled thinking.

Suddenly Luis was frozen with fear. He got the cold sweats. That young man in the red shirt was coming towards him with two big policemen in front of him. Usually the cops looked the other way when they saw us luckers. The red shirted young man said, "There he is officers. He is scaring customers."

Victor's voice boomed like on a public-address system in this place. "Luis. You dumb ass! I told you to stay out of trouble. Now you got to cut and run."

Luis got even more confused. He knew he couldn't out-run the cops with his cart so he grabbed for the knife. The cops started shouting for him to drop it and put his hands on his head. Luis's thinking got real jumbled. Did the red shirted young man know big Red? Victor was saying nothing now. Victor had last told Luis to cut and run. Luis decided he had to cut his way out first, then, he could run fast with his new cart. As he moved toward the officers their guns went off with a huge roar. The bullets hit Luis's chest. A terrible pain struck him. Then as Luis's vision grew rapidly dim he had a last picture of his beloved Sister Laura. She had no smile, only a stark look of fear, then sadness just before the darkness.

A tearful Sister Laura was the only one attending Luis's graveside funeral. She said a prayer for Luis's recently departed soul and then reading a poem out loud.

LUIS

Hear a disheveled lovable man

of the restless street corners,

and shabby lives under bridges.

> This frightened unsmiling city,
>
> blinded by the neon gloom
>
> of endless allies soon forgotten.
>
> Hear lonely souls unredeemed,
>
> and homeless in the streets.

Sadly, tragically, Luis never had psychotherapy.

LESSONS LEARNED FROM LUIS

Clergy like Sister Laura make efforts to provide God's love in a world that is often cruel and compassionless. Sometimes though, love is not enough. Psychotherapy and pharmacotherapy for severely chronically mentally ill homeless persons is available at over-burdened public clinics. But, active teams to reach out to these folks are expensive and challenging to sustain. Such work has a high risk of burnout. Such teams' successes do occur, but are often go unheralded.

8—A BOY WHO LOVED HIS CRAZY DAD

"My dad and I hunt bugs. Bugs hide in goofy places. My dad's apartment is fun. When I stay at dad's we play FBI guys. Cockroaches can carry little cameras and tape-recorders. When dad and I go to the zoo or the park we have fun. When we get home, we check for those bugs. Even tiny ants need to be found and killed. Thing is—we don't often find those bugs. But, it is fun looking for them with dad." Davey Scott 9 years old.

****

Tom Tolman MD drove toward the Houston VA Hospital in his silver gray MGB. He called it Silver B and enjoyed driving with the top down. The fall day is clear and cool. Tolman enjoys his part-time work at the VA Hospital. Today he is seeing patients at the day hospital. The day hospital is a small freestanding unit for out-patients who have recently been in-patients or those sent from the out-patient clinic for daily treatment to prevent the need for acute hospitalization. Tolman's first appointment was with the ex-wife of a patient in daily treatment. The nurse at the day hospital said that Wanda Scott was demanding to see a doctor immediately.

The slender, dark-haired woman waiting to see Tom had a perpetual frown wrinkling her otherwise pretty face. The scent of overly pungent perfume preceded her and her provocatively tight sweater and pants clamored for attention.

Wanda Scott was clearly distraught. She dispensed with any pleasantries and blurted out the reason for her distress. "Doctor, you can't let my son Davey spend weekends all alone with Howard, he's too crazy. He's dangerous, too dangerous to take care of Davey by himself."

"Mrs. Scott, I will see and examine your ex-husband this morning and decide what the situation requires."

"Look Dr. Tolman, my nine-year-old son, Davey, and I are doing fine. I have a with job at Walmart and get a portion of Howard's VA benefits check. Howard has spent time with Davey but only during a few weekend days when he's been chaperoned by a Methodist minister friend of mine. Now Howard wants to take Davey to his cheap apartment for the whole weekend. I am dead set against that idea. You better not let crazy Howard take Davey for weekends. If you do, I will get an attorney."

They didn't cover this situation in the textbooks I read. Guess I must become Solomon to tackle this one.

****

Howard Scott was chronically suspicious and occasionally appeared to hallucinate and suffer mild delusions. Those episodes were infrequent and never violent in nature. Howard talked about ways he would silence the voices using poetry-writing and music. Howard shared with the group his thoughts that CIA agents wanted him to spy for them and keep watch for communist agents. The agents were, he said, trying to get information about VA patients like him who had served in the Vietnam War so the United States would not lose another war like the lost war in Vietnam. Even when another patient occasionally confronted Howard in group about his contentions, Howard would smile and say things like, "You don't fully understand buddy."

Before seeing Howard, Tolman consulted with Howard's group therapist and the psychiatry resident who was prescribing Howard's antipsychotic medications. Both agreed that

Howard had made a good recovery from a psychotic episode that had required hospitalization three months ago. Howard had, in fact, done so well that he was actively looking for a job.

Tolman invited Howard to sit down with his cup of coffee. He leaned back in his chair as he sipped from the Styrofoam cup. Howard was about five-feet-nine and slender. He spoke clearly without any disordered thinking except the one area about his suspicions about Communists. That preoccupation was like an isolated private concern that almost seemed like an old war buddy. Howard had lost friends in Vietnam and said he finally was working on his grief about lost war buddies in his current group therapy. It had taken him a long time to trust the group but he valued it now and wouldn't miss a session.

Tolman told Howard about his ex-wife's concern. Howard said, "Dr. Tolman, Wanda is a good woman. I still love her. She loves Davey like I do. Probably more. Wanda just couldn't deal with my stress and fear spells. Since she got the divorce she seems more comfortable when we see each other. Wanda seems bossy all the time since I got out of the hospital. Her daddy died in San Antonio state hospital.

"I tried to explain to Wanda that when my meds are dialed-in right I can sleep good and I don't get up-tight. The meds don't make me like a zombie like they did at first. Even when I was the most up-tight I never thought about hurting anyone. The only time I hurt and killed people was when I was in uniform in Vietnam. I wouldn't ever hurt Davey."

Tolman said, "Howard, I would like to visit with Davey and want to suggest that Wanda meet with one of our social workers here at day hospital. That would allow her to let us know about her concerns and learn more about therapy and being a single parent."

Howard thought about the plan and wanted to know when he could see Davey for weekends. Tolman said he would tell him the decision after he had seen Davey. Howard agreed with the plan.

****

Davey Scott was skinny and had black hair and brown eyes like his dad. He had a mischievous grin in a Huck Finn/Tom Sawyer style. Davey had special interest in the brain demonstration model that Tolman had on his desk and asked, "Dr. Tolman, is that the way my brain looks inside? Can you tell me where dreams are found in there?"

Tolman explained the brain model and pointed out some of the brain regions that are involved with the dream experience. Tom also said that dreams help us solve problems and can help us understand our feelings. When Tom asked Davey about his dreams, Davey replied, "I dreamed about trying to find a puppy that my friend, who lives next door, had lost. I also had dreams about seeing my dad in a hospital a long time ago. In those dreams dad was smiling and waving to me from the window of his hospital room."

Davey was happy to visit with his dad at pastor Wentworth's church recently. "We played together on the church's kids' play area. I wish I could visit dad at his apartment. Dad says there's a city swimming pool nearby.

Tolman told Davey he would see him again and that he would recommend to his mother that he should be able to visit with his dad on weekends twice a month. Davey seemed very happy with that.

Tolman was pleased and relieved that Wanda Scott had agreed to meet weekly with a day hospital social worker named Star Davis. Wanda was wary about Tolman's plan but after some reassurances agreed to Davey visiting with Howard at his apartment twice a month. Wanda would alert Star if she detected any problems.

The visitation program went well. Howard and Davey enjoyed swimming, movies, and visiting the Houston Zoo and the museums around Herman Park. Howard patiently helped Davey with his homework. Wanda reported her pleasant surprise that Davey was doing even better in school.

Several months later Howard had a significant setback requiring hospitalization. Howard with the help of his group therapist spotted the early symptoms of his relapsing schizoaffective condition. Howard himself called Wanda to cancel visits until his treatment succeeded. Howard also explained the situation to Davey who told Howard that he would pray for him to get better quickly. Howard was touched and told his therapy group that Davey's prayers motivated him to get through the depressive episode as soon as it was possible.

The episode involved a severe depression around Easter, which was the occasion of Howard's first psychotic episode when he was in his early twenties. Easter was often a tough time for Howard. Star Davis helped Wanda to understand Howard's condition and even discussed the increased possibility that Davey might someday experience depression. Wanda read a lot of material about the genetic aspects of depression and became involved with the Houston Bipolar Disorder Association.

LESSONS LEARNED FROM DAVEY SCOTT AND HIS DAD

Tom Tolman's notes:

It is heartening and encouraging when group and individual psychotherapy is successful. Such is not always the case. Chronic severe mental illness isn't automatically associated with defective parenting. The love and prayers of a resilient little boy like Davey Scott for the "crazy" dad he loves is touching and inspiring. Such situations make psychiatry work wonderfully worthwhile at times.

www.ingramcontent.com/pod-product-compliance
Lightning Source LLC
Chambersburg PA
CBHW071220220526
45468CB00002B/686